BEAUTY MATTERS

How to Be a Fabulous Woman? Improve Your Self Confidence, Discover Beauty Secrets, and Learn Our "Without Surgery" Approaches to Find the Beauty Hidden in You

Beauty Matters

Table Of Contents

Introduction

Beauty is one of a woman's most essential traits. It sets them apart from the rest and is one of the first things you notice about someone. There are different tips to be the fabulous woman you are looking for. If you're looking for a quick fix, buy yourself some new clothes, get a touch-up at the salon or get a manicure. But if you have time, try some of these tips to improve your natural beauty: improve your posture; eat healthy meals and snacks regularly; avoid excess calories and sugar whenever possible; drink plenty of water every day; exercise regularly to maintain muscle tone and skin that doesn't sag from lack of use or elasticity.

But there is more than one way to define beauty: it is not only found on the outside, but also on the inside. We all have our quirks and flaws; learning to find inner peace takes work, but yields great benefits. If you want to be more beautiful, you must increase your idea or concept of what beauty is. Many people will disagree with this, but it is true.

Everyone has a different understanding of beauty. For some, it is something that can be easily defined with the perfect set of features and absolute mastery of makeup. For others, beauty is a feeling or a choice. However, one thing we can all agree on is that being beautiful doesn't have to be about looking good for someone else, sometimes it's about looking good for yourself. But who says being confident in yourself has to come at a cost? Sometimes it comes with the package. We all have days when we start to feel like we're never good enough, and the effects can be brutal. Sometimes doubting yourself can be worth it, because beauty isn't always about how you look...it's about how you feel when you put your face on every morning. When your skin goes from flaky and dry to moisturized and beautiful, that's what beauty is really all about.

A beautiful person will always look attractive no matter what they wear or how much makeup they put on; this is because they take care of themselves and radiate positivity. Also, keep in mind that people don't refer to themselves as insecure or ugly; no one wants to be called less than beautiful because it makes them feel unimportant and unappreciated.

While some people may be born with everything they need to be physically attractive, others need to work on it little by little until they can create their own perfect image, which is what everyone is looking for inside.

Some women think that taking care of their appearance is a waste of time and that it is something reserved only for superficial women with a lot of free time. I think these women are actually just afraid to dare. Taking care of ourselves and getting to know ourselves, improving our appearance is a great act of love for ourselves. Looking in the mirror and appreciating our image is very important for our self-esteem. The danger is when someone looks for perfection that does not exist. I just want to teach you to appreciate your strengths, because I'm sure you have many more than you think.

In this book, you will learn the different "beauty without surgery" tips to adopt in your daily life, as well as things that will help you improve your self-esteem. Whether you are looking for tips on how to do your makeup, go natural, or just want some emerging ideas on what to do with your hair for that special occasion, we assure you that you will find more confidence in yourself and discover the inner and outer beauty that hides inside you.

CHAPTER 1:

Your Diet:
How Your Diet Affects Your Beauty

The right diet for beauty is, well, the perfect diet. And it's not just because eating a balanced diet can prevent chronic disease and promote overall wellness. It's because doing so can result in skin that glows with radiance and a glowing smile to match. Here are some dietary tips that work:

- The best way to get the nutrients from fresh fruits and vegetables is to consume them raw or in juice form. This way, you get the maximum health benefits without cooking out the toxins in the food by heating it above 115 degrees Fahrenheit (46 degrees Celsius).

- A diet rich in vitamin C and wild salmon, rich in omega-3 fatty acids, helps improve dry skin by keeping it supple.

- Daily consumption of a major source of zinc, such as oysters or pumpkin seeds, helps reduce acne-promoting hormone levels. Topical zinc is also practical: just apply a zinc cream to the skin for best results.

- Eating right keeps you looking fresh and glowing. If you eat a diet rich in fruits, vegetables, whole grains, and lean proteins, you'll have the vitamins you need for beautiful skin from the inside out.

- Consuming plenty of calcium-rich foods, such as calcium-fortified juices and yogurts, will give you more calcium than you could get from a pill. Calcium has been shown to reduce the amount of skin pigmentation in adults over the age of 20. It also helps strengthen bones in children ages 9 to 18.

- Fresh vegetables are also excellent sources of these nutrients, especially for overall health, but you can get more overall by juicing them fresh. Juices rich in vitamins A, C, and E are excellent sources of antioxidants that help fight free radicals that can damage skin cells.

Benefits of Hydration

When you are hot, it doesn't take long for your skin or hair to dry out. This can happen if you spend too much time in the sun or if the air is too dry, which is especially common in winter. You should keep your body hydrated for both hair and skin.

A very effective way to keep your skin looking its best is to drink plenty of water. And how much? Well, for healthy skin, you should aim to consume 2 liters (approximately 8 glasses) every day. Keep in mind that while coffee and tea can also provide some hydration, they are not good for the skin; we'll talk about that later in this article.

Drinking water can do more than just keep your skin soft and supple. Drinking enough water can also help you lose weight. When you drink water, your body does several things:

It signals your brain that you are full, so you eat less. It helps flush waste out of your body, which makes your skin look cleaner and healthier. The body uses it to eliminate toxins, and toxins create acne. It strengthens the immune system, making you less prone to ailments.

One of the most important factors in having beautiful skin is making sure your body gets enough water. It is important to note that drinking coffee, tea, or soda does not count towards your daily water intake. These drinks will hydrate you, but they probably won't help you keep your skin looking good.

How Alcoholism Affects Your Beauty?

Going out for a drink? Have you ever wondered if drinking alcohol is bad for your beauty? There are many ways alcohol can affect your appearance.

Dehydration

Alcohol naturally dehydrates the body. The stomach, which normally produces hydrochloric acid, does not produce enough of this substance when alcohol is consumed. As a result, the body has to increase saliva production to compensate for this because alcohol is irritating. Increased saliva production can lead to mouth ulcers and dry mouth over time.

Aging

Collagen is a protein that keeps our skin smooth and firm. Collagen also keeps our nails strong and prevents them from splitting. Alcohol breaks down collagen fibers, which causes wrinkles in the skin, known as "aging" of the face. Long-term alcohol consumption can also lead to premature aging or even loss of facial hair or nails, as collagen also serves as a building block for hair and nails.

Acne

Alcohol can cause skin problems such as acne. Acne is triggered when skin pores become clogged with dead skin cells or oil. Alcohol is notorious for clogging pores, which can make them appear larger and more noticeable. Drinking too much can lead to dry skin, as water is also drawn out of the body from other areas as excess fluid leaves the body as a result of excessive alcohol consumption.

Hair Loss

Alcohol has many detrimental effects on hair. If you have been drinking, you have been drawing water out of your body, which will cause the body to start losing all the nutrients it needs to nourish the hair and skin from the foods you eat. This will induce a deficit, which will result in hair loss.

Benefits of Oils

Beauty is a way of expressing individuality, and it is a deep-seated need in every human being. Here are some healthy oils that will give your skin a youthful glow.

Olive oil contains therapeutic antioxidants that can help keep skin smooth, silky, and elastic. It also helps diminish the appearance of wrinkles by encouraging cell regeneration in the connective structure of the skin.

Mineral oil is another fantastic option for moisturizing dry skin, as it helps retain suppleness by locking moisture into the skin. Almond oil also contains vitamin A, which can help in the treatment of acne and blemishes.

These natural oils are the perfect choice to keep your skin looking healthy and glowing. If you use them regularly, you will notice a significant difference in your skin and how it looks and feels.

Benefits of Vitamin E

Vitamin E has been shown to fight free radicals and is known for its antioxidant and anti-inflammatory properties. The vitamin also reduces both sun damage and signs of aging, as recent studies have shown. Vitamin E has anti-inflammatory properties and also helps reduce sun damage to the skin,

There are many forms of vitamin E, which affects its effectiveness. Alpha-tocopherol is a natural form of vitamin E found in plants and fruits. It is a very effective antioxidant for skin protection. Vitamin E can also be found in small amounts in avocado, sunflower seeds, and wheat germ oil. The recommended dose of vitamin E is 2 to 3 grams per day.

CHAPTER 2:

Your Posture

The posture of a woman is one of the most significant and beautiful aspects of her elegance.

Good posture will make any figure more attractive. Proportionate body measurements are very important, but if your posture is poor, even perfect figures and shapes will be destroyed. Poor posture is your worst enemy. Your posture, the way you walk, sit, stand, and move can make or break the way you look. If you behave like a kangaroo, slouch like a camel and act like a hyena, no one will remember your fancy dress or accessories!

Often, the most important thing is not what you weigh, but the way you carry yourself, the way you present yourself, your body language, etc. I have seen some women with excess fat and less than perfect figures walk and stand, sit and stand gracefully, and in doing so look so elegant and attractive. These women become living proof that good posture is a definite and most important requirement for feeling and looking more attractive.

Designer clothes or the latest accessories are useless if your posture is undesirable. Poor posture makes a woman look ordinary and insignificant.

Work to improve your posture because it has a direct bearing not only on your beauty but also on your health.

Thin women with poor posture, tall girls with a curved spine and slumped shoulders, short women crawl around like little bears or like kangaroos craning their necks or like little ducks to look taller, wear heels that are too big to add extra inches and, in the bargain, defeat the very purpose of looking taller by drawing all the attention to their short stature and poor posture. They look ridiculous.

A woman of short stature looks much better in medium heels for regular wear and even looks taller and poised. Save the high heels/stilettos for occasions, such as formal parties where you don't have to walk much. It is inexcusable for any healthy woman to have poor posture. You need to do everything you can to improve it. If you cannot or will not work on improving your posture, please do not spend your time with this program as, before we move on to other topics to improve your appearance, we need to concentrate on posture. A human being is meant to move like a human being - that is how nature intended us, humans, to move. So if you have a bad posture, you have to work hard to improve it, and there is no other way; there are no shortcuts. Good posture is very important, and that's final. Nobody can help you if you can't work to improve your posture.

Your whole image will change in a short 3 weeks (at most), and that is guaranteed. However, it requires diligent attention and practice as much as anything else. It is up to you to decide if you want to pay attention to this aspect. Remember that you are helping yourself and no one else. So do yourself a favor and, first and foremost, watch your posture. If it's ugly, do whatever it takes to work on improving it. The easiest and most effective way is to become aware of your posture all the time; you can do this by being conscious of your body's alignment, at first you will have to constantly remind yourself of it, but as the days go by it will become natural and you will start to be aware of it until one fine day, about three weeks of conscious effort, your posture will have improved considerably. Keep at it. Don't give up, and you will be pleasantly surprised by the results.

Did you know that your mood affects your posture? Present yourself in a way that the world believes in you, and you will begin to believe in yourself. Mood and awareness are what you need to increase your poise. For example: If you look poised, you will begin to feel poised. No matter how beautiful you look, you will not get others to believe you are beautiful if your posture is not right. Learn to put on your assets and believe deep down inside that you are beautiful.

Be conscious of your movements at first until you feel comfortable with your new "moves".

Practicing Good Posture

Good body alignment! What is this? It's nothing but your posture. It's the way you carry yourself. Proper body alignment is a straight line from your head to your shoulders, down to your hips, and ending at your feet.

Here are some tips to correct your body alignment:

- Bring the ears back over your shoulders.

- Keep your chin parallel to the floor.

- Keep your shoulders down and relaxed

- Elevate your rib cage.

- Stomach – pull it in and keep it taut at all times.

- Pelvis – tuck it in and tilt it slightly forward. (Will make you look sexier!)

- Knees – relax them and keep them flexed.

- Feet – let your weight fall on the center of your feet.

- Exercise and stretch your body to strengthen your full back muscles as well as your abdominal muscles. These are the muscles that support a great posture!

Don't strike stiff, artificial poses or take really ugly steps. If you make an exaggerated effort to look poised, it shows, it's unattractive; it's as ugly as bad posture. So the trick is to get comfortable with your new body alignment awareness techniques until you show ease in trusting your posture to yourself, and that only comes with practice and self-awareness.

If you carry yourself gracefully, no matter how much you weigh or how tall or short or average you are, if you carry yourself gracefully, you will look and feel more attractive. It doesn't matter how carefully you choose your clothes, or how expensive your dresses and accessories are, or even if the best designer designs your clothes: if you lack grace and confidence in your body, nothing can make up for it. On the other hand, the woman who carries herself with grace and confidence can make even the cheapest and most ordinary outfit look stunning.

Controlling Your Weight!

It's simple, if you are overweight, you need to eat sensibly and exercise to burn off the excess weight. You have to work towards an attractive figure by exercising regularly, and you have to follow a balanced, self-controlled diet. There are no magic potions: exercising and eating a proper diet is the only way to lose excess weight and have a slim figure; it is easy to incorporate this healthy habit into your life when you realize the benefits you can gain in your overall health and fitness by following this regimen. If you are underweight, you should also exercise and follow a nutritious, balanced diet to reach your desired healthy weight. (More on this later).

Tip: A low-carbohydrate diet (especially low in wheat) helps. Eliminating sugar and processed foods also helps. Increasing protein in the diet helps. Increasing fiber and drinking enough water to hydrate from within.

CHAPTER 3:

Your Hygiene: Overview

What is Personal Hygiene?

Personal hygiene is a set of practices to keep us clean and healthy. It usually refers to the practices of bathing, shampooing, cleaning teeth, and other hygiene practices. It includes the opposite extremes of hygiene: sanitary practices that prevent or reduce disease and disease transmission in the school environment, hygiene that reduces the risk of infection, such as handwashing with soap for effective prevention of diarrhea. It also incorporates personal appearance with emphasis on clothing choices and personal grooming habits.

Personal hygiene and beauty are important factors for the body and mind. This is especially true for women, who tend to think of themselves in physical terms and rate their attractiveness on a scale. Our personal hygiene is something we should be proud of because it affects not only our body but also our health. Self-care helps us feel confident about ourselves, which promotes positive mental health.

Different Types of Hygiene

Here are some of the standard Hygiene Practices:

Hair Hygiene

Hygienic Hair practices include hair washing and conditioning, dandruff, and other hair treatments.

Nail Hygiene

Nail Hygiene includes cutting our nails, manicure/pedicure, or cleaning our nails at least twice a week.

Skin and Body Hygiene

Body Hygiene includes taking a bath, applying deodorant, and many other remedies to fight body odor.

Mental Hygiene

Even our brain needs hygiene by making sure it is staying hydrated and nourished. Proper diet usually affects the way we think and memorize.

Oral Hygiene

Oral hygiene includes flossing and brushing our teeth and other dental care practices to keep your teeth from any problems and potential loss in the future.

Feminine Hygiene

Feminine hygiene simply means maintaining intimate health. It is one of the essential hygiene regimens for women. Feminine hygiene includes sanitary protection through the use of tampons, pads, and panty liners. Feminine hygiene is more concerned with the care and cleanliness of a woman's private parts. In other words, it involves the use of personal care products by women during menstruation.

As the adage goes, cleanliness is next to godliness. Neglecting hygiene can cause health and social problems that you may not even be aware of. Problems like dandruff are forgivable, but good looks are often the result of attention to grooming. If you want to look fabulous and great every day, you need to put some work and time into your hygiene.

CHAPTER 4:

Your Hygiene:
Cleaning Your Face And Body

I t is time to turn our attention to how we can preserve, protect and keep our skin looking young and beautiful. The first tool we have to preserve the youthfulness of our skin is our skin cleansing practice. Although cleansing is simple and easy to understand, there are some aspects of our cleansing routines that we have been doing incorrectly for years. In this chapter, we will first look at how we cleanse our skin and then take a look at the individual components and our cleansing routine to understand why. In doing so, you will have both the knowledge of how to cleanse and why in this specific way.

How to Clean Your Skin?

Remember to find out what skin type you have. The reason we want this information is so we can get the most out of our skincare routine by tailoring it to our skin type. For example, while it is recommended that you wash your skin twice a day, it is also recommended that those with dry skin consider washing their face less frequently. Similarly, people with oily skin may consider washing their face two or possibly three times a day, depending on how oily their skin is.

Before washing your face, wash your hands with soap and warm water. This serves to remove germs from your hands and any dirt that may have accumulated during the day before washing. Since one of the main reasons we wash our face is to remove dirt and germ buildup, if we don't wash our hands, we are exposing our face to more germs when we clean it.

Wash your face twice a day with warm water instead of hot water. A good time to clean your face is when you wake up and before you go to bed. When you wake up, you've been asleep for eight hours, which is plenty of time for germs and dirt to get on your face. It's a good idea to wash when you wake up to prevent them from staying on your skin longer than necessary. Likewise, when you wash your skin in the evening, you'll be removing the day's dirt so it doesn't go untreated for another eight hours. If you wear makeup, be sure to remove it before washing your face or going to bed.

Using warm water, gently massage your face with your fingers. Instead of scrubbing your skin, use slow, circular motions. Avoid overworking or mistreating the skin around the eyes, as this is the most fragile area of the face. You can exfoliate your skin; however, this process can be harmful to those with sensitive skin or those who have acne or other skin problems.

Once the cleansing is complete, it is time to rinse your face. This should be done with lukewarm water, either with a cool washcloth or by cupping your hands together and splashing it on your face. This step is doubly important if you exfoliated your skin or used products during your cleansing ritual, as these products can clog your pores and cause irritation or blemishes when they stay on your skin. Next, you should dry your freshly cleansed skin. It is important to pat your skin dry rather than rubbing it.

How to Clean Your Body?

To cleanse the body, you should shower once a day. Although some sources recommend baths, it's best to shower, as baths are more likely to leach out natural moisturizing oils and can be especially damaging to your skin if yours is drier. But by showering, you remove the bacteria that cause body odor as well as the dirt and grime that can clog your pores.

While showering, use your hands to clean your body. You can be tougher on your body compared to your face. Using your hands is a cleaner solution than resorting to scouring pads or other cleansers; studies have shown that these cleaning tools build up bacteria quickly and can damage your skin by exposing it to more threats. Your hands are a much better tool. Bar soap or body wash is fine to use on your body, as these don't see the same buildup of dangerous bacteria as scouring pads. If you exfoliate your body, you should only do it once a week, and even then, you should only focus on acne-prone areas. Excessive exfoliation will irritate the skin and even worsen any acne problems you have.

It is a good habit to pat your body dry instead of brushing or scrubbing. Body skin is not as sensitive as facial skin, but it can still cause damage if dried incorrectly. Stay in a steamy bath while you dry off, as the steam will help open your pores and moisturize your skin.

Avoid Using Generic Bar Soap on Your Face

Since the skin on the body is tougher than the skin on the face, using bar soap on the body is perfectly acceptable. But using bar soap on the face is a bad idea, as these soaps can upset the pH balance of the skin. This means they can alter the skin on the face so that bacteria and yeast have an easier time growing. One of the key goals of skincare is to avoid exposing the skin and pores to harmful bacteria, so using bar soap on the face is not good.

Foaming soaps can also strip the skin of the natural oils needed to keep it healthy. A 2012 study found that surfactants in foaming soap can cause skin molecules to become disorganized. When the molecules are in order, the skin looks natural and healthy, so if you want to keep your skin beautiful, you should avoid any disruption in the order of its molecules. It is better to use your hands to clean your face than a bar of soap.

Use Lukewarm Water Instead of Hot Water

There is a myth that has circulated for years. Pores are similar to doors. Cold water closes pores while hot water opens them. Although it's a catchy rhyme, this myth is not true. Never use water so hot that it leaves your skin red. The negative effects of using water that is too hot are further exacerbated on days when the air is dry. This behavior can cause or exacerbate acne breakouts.

Avoid Using Wipes, Especially If They Are Shared

It is advisable to pat the skin dry, whether it is the skin on the face or the rest of the body. This is because when you use a wipe, what you are doing is a scrubbing motion. This motion pulls on the skin and can scratch the protective barrier that makes up the top layer. Damaging this layer impairs the skin's ability to protect itself from harmful bacteria and irritates the skin, which can worsen problems such as acne or breakouts.

By patting the skin dry, the motion no longer pulls on the skin, so it no longer scratches the surface and damages that protective layer. Instead, you're removing water in a way that respects the skin and ensures it remains as healthy as possible. Even if you think the water will hydrate your skin, it may actually cause dryness when it evaporates. It's important to dry your skin, but make sure you dry it properly.

Every time you wash your face, if you're not careful to wash your hands first, you expose your face to bacteria on your person. When you share a washcloth, you increase the number of bacteria you expose yourself to, because you are not only dealing with bacteria coming off of you, but also bacteria coming from someone else. Always use a clean towel and never share it with others.

Avoid Over-Washing

When you wash your face too often, you damage your skin by stripping it of the natural oils that keep it healthy. The proper amount of washes per day should never be more than three, and most people will want to wash their face only twice a day for best results.

Remember that when you shower, you are most likely washing your face as well. So, if you shower when you wake up in the morning and wash your face during that shower, you don't need to follow up with a specific face wash. Instead, count your shower as your morning wash and go about your day. It's better to err on the side of caution and wash only twice than to overdo it and damage your skin.

Avoid Washing Too Long

As with over-washing the face, washing for too long also damages the skin's protective layer. We leave the water on the skin for longer than necessary and cleanse too vigorously, which causes more pulling on the skin and more damage.

You should never wash your face for more than one minute. This is enough time to reach all the crevices of the face and ensure a thorough wash. If you go over one minute, you are over-washing and putting your skin's health at risk.

CHAPTER 5:

Your Skin:
Understanding Your Skin Type

The skin is the largest organ of our body, and we are curious that it is our body's first line of defense. It is a really important topic for our beauty, that's why I have dedicated six chapters to it. The skin is our identity card and it shows how old we are, whether we smoke or not, if we are sufficiently hydrated, if we do enough exercise. Our skin also affects the way we see ourselves with confidence. In addition, the skin helps regulate our body temperature and protects us from the sun, etc.

The 5 Common Skin Types

How important is it to know your skin type? It is important to know your skin type because each person's skin is special, and knowing it allows you to take proper care of it. Knowing your skin type allows you to choose the right products for your skin. Also, knowing your skin type helps you prepare your skin for makeup products, and if you prefer not to apply makeup at all, proper skincare will allow you to do without it. Knowing your skin type is efficient and cost-effective because you won't have to buy what you don't need.

Dry Skin

Dry skin is caused by inadequate sebum production, which results in a lack of oil. As I said earlier, women's sebum production decreases as they age. You should know that genetics can cause dry skin. Cold season and winter are external factors that cause dry skin due to lack of moisture. Showering for a long time causes dry skin. It could be the reason why some people shower less frequently. Keep in mind that showering is part of hygiene; hygiene is part of having healthy skin, so you might decide to shower often and spend less time in the shower. How do we identify dry skin? Is it flaky, feels tight, dull, lacks oil, and can lead to premature aging. The way to care for dry skin is to frequently apply moisturizers, serums, and facial masks. Drinking enough water also helps to keep it hydrated. Cleansing the skin during the wet season can be helpful, and applying toners would balance the pH of the skin.

Oily Skin

This is the overproduction of the sebaceous gland that causes the skin to develop acne and breakouts. Oily skin is caused by having large pores. Genetics may be one of the causes of oily skin. People who live in a tropical or humid climate are more likely to have oily skin. Hormonal imbalances in women during pregnancy or the menstrual cycle can cause excess sebum production resulting in acne breakouts. Men are more prone to acne because their body produces more sebum and they have larger pores. Therefore, they are prone to clogged pores and acne. In addition, frequent exfoliation can irritate the skin and cause it to produce more sebum. Women produce less sebum than men after puberty.

How do we identify oily skin? It has enlarged pores, is more likely to have blackheads and blemishes, and a very shiny appearance around the T-zone due to excess sebaceous glands. You should know that people with oily skin tend to age more slowly than people with dry skin.

Normal Skin

Normal skin has balanced pH and sebum levels. Normal skin does not become too oily or too dry. The way to identify normal skin is that it has an even skin tone, very smooth, balanced sebaceous glands, and no open pores. Normal skin is very moisturized. The way to care for normal skin is to follow a simple skincare routine that keeps it hydrated and healthy.

Mixed Skin

People with this skin type have oil around the T-zone, on the nose, and forehead. They have dry cheeks and eyes. This is common because environmental factors trigger it. You should know that the use of aggressive products causes combination skin to experience acne on the nose and chin. The way to take care of this skin is to establish a daily skincare routine and get products that are gentle on the skin.

Sensitive Skin

This skin type reacts to everything, environmental conditions, free radicals, skincare, and even clothing. The way you know you have sensitive skin is that your skin reacts to skin products. Long hours in the shower cause it to redden, and when it reacts to tight clothing, the sensations are itchy. Skin texture is fine and prone to broken capillaries. The skin feels flaky and dry during cold or winter seasons, and moisturizing is the only way to keep the skin happy. During the summer, the opposite is true, as the skin becomes so oily that you need to apply less moisturizer and focus more on sun protection. This type of skin can be expensive because you have to buy gentle or organic products, and maintaining it means not using what everyone else is using, as it might not work for you.

How to Determine Your Skin Type?

Any licensed dermatologist will tell you how important it is to choose skincare products based on your skin type. If the product is not right for you, it will not work as well and may cause skin defections/reactions. So before you buy a moisturizer, cleanser, or anything else for your skin, you should first determine your skin type.

The amount of oil and water in your skin determines your skin type. Your skin will suffer if it is out of balance. For example, if your skin is too oily, you may be more prone to acne breakouts and your skin will look shiny. Oily skincare products are oil-free and may contain ingredients that help rebalance the skin's oil level.

Another common problem is dry skin, which is caused by a lack of water in the skin and leads to itching and tightness; dry skin appears visibly flaky and can even cause fine lines. Products designed for dry skin are usually water-based to add much-needed moisture to the skin. It is also possible to have combination skin, which means that some areas of the face are oily and others are dry. People with this skin type can use products for combination skin or use different products on different areas of the face.

Finally, there is normal skin, which has the right balance of oil and water. Some people can tell their skin type by looking in the mirror. Others can tell if they have dry, oily, or normal skin; on the other hand, if you are unsure of your skin type, you should see a dermatologist. Make sure you only use products that are suitable for your skin type.

There are several ways to identify your skin:

- If your skin is smooth and free of imperfections, with no greasy or dry patches, you have normal skin! Other signs of normal skin include small, barely visible pores and the absence of breakouts. It is very little to no sensitivity.

- Dry skin is defined as rough, flaky, or tight. Pores are almost imperceptible, as are dry or red patches and visible fine lines.

- You have oily skin if it appears and feels shiny, greasy, and/or slippery.

- Combination skin is both the best and the worst of both worlds.

It is usually characterized by an oily T-zone (on the forehead and nose) and dry or normal skin on the rest of the face. The pores on the nose and possibly the forehead are enlarged, but smaller on the rest of the facial skin, which may be shiny, especially around the T-zone. Climate and time can make the combination skin dry and flaky at times, but oily and prone to acne breakouts at others.

CHAPTER 6:

Your Skin: Daily Skincare Basics

O ur skin becomes our first outfit, and it needs a little attention, but that doesn't mean we all have to be scientists. A few good habits with your daily routine... and you'll see the benefits. A routine is the foundation of everything, and if you stick to it, you can set your skin up for life. In the morning and evening, 2-3 minutes for your skin, or longer if you want it to be more relaxing. A good skincare routine is not judged by the number of different products you use or the number of steps you follow. One or two products complete with a cleanser and sunscreen in the morning and one or two additional products for the evening, and there you go to bed for clearer, better skin in the morning.

Yes, it's interesting that the basic skincare regimen takes a few minutes - and that's it!

<u>Cleansing</u>

A good cleansing routine keeps your skin healthy, naturally glowing, and protected from diseases.

The skin is your first line of defense against environmental toxins and pollutants that can disrupt its functioning. Cleansing the skin will not only remove all that dirt we pick up from day to night, but it will also remove sun damage, microorganisms, and the damage we deliberately cause by applying various anti-aging and other luxury products. There is a wide range of cleansing products on the market, such as bar soaps, foaming, and non-foaming cleansers, toners, exfoliators, cleansing oils and milks, and micellar water, but skin type, budget, and personal preferences are what decide which product is right for you.

Bar Soaps

Bar soaps are usually not as gentle on delicate skin, such as facial skin. They can strip essential oil or lipids from the top layer of skin, leaving the skin barrier compromised. This causes accelerated water loss, resulting in dull, dehydrated skin. People with dry and sensitive skin should avoid cleansing with bars of soap. People with oily skin can use them frequently.

Non-Foaming and Foaming Cleansers

Non-foaming cleansers, good for dry or sensitive skin type, are gentler and do not foam when mixed with water. While foaming cleansers, good for oily skin, produce foam when wet. These cleansers may not be the ideal choice for many people because they can leave residue on the skin.

Cleansing Toners

One of the most popular cleansers is toners that are used to cleanse with a cotton pad instead of water. Toners are alcohol-based and cleanse dirt and oil effectively, but are usually used after cleansing. Toners work well on oily and acne-prone skin, but can sometimes cause irritation and dryness.

Cleansing Milk

Like the toner, cleansing milk is also used to cleanse with a cotton pad rather than water. Cleansing milk leaves moisturizing agents on the skin that help heal the skin barrier and moisturize the skin.

Facial Oils or Balms

Facial oils work well for all skin types. Cleansing with oil is a gentle way to remove makeup and SPF, especially for sensitive skin. These oils help protect the lipid layer and the good bacteria that live on the skin. It is best to use a facial oil suitable for your skin type that dissolves well and nourishes the skin.

Micellar Waters

Micellar waters have gained a lot of popularity in recent years. They are good for all skin types, including oily skin. The tiny micelles in the water remove dirt and impurities from the skin. However, they should not be used as a primary source of cleansing.

Serum

A serum is a product that delivers a high concentration of specific active ingredients directly to the skin. You should choose a serum with active ingredients that can help treat the condition of your skin. The serum is applied before the moisturizer.

Facial serums are usually water-based, clear, gel-like solutions with concentrated efficacy. When applied to the face, the small molecules are absorbed in a short time to penetrate deep into the skin. Serums (and essences, very similar to serums) are rich in concentrated active ingredients such as vitamins, antioxidants, peptides, and more that are good for reducing dryness, dark spots, uneven skin tone, and fine lines. Serums are great for all skin types, but you should use the one that is appropriate for your skin type and the skin problem you want to treat.

Only a few drops of serum are needed. Apply the serum with your fingertips and let it absorb for at least five minutes before moving on to the next step in your skincare routine: moisturizing.

Moisturizing

This is the last moisturizing step in your routine before going for SPF.

Moisturizers are a must for maintaining the elasticity of the top layer of skin, as they help improve its texture making it more supple and well hydrated.

Moisturizers are generally classified into three categories:

- **Emollients**

These add oil to the epidermis to soften the skin and are found in dry skin products. Emollients include ceramides, linoleic acid, dimethicone, and capryloylglycol, to name a few.

- **Humectants**

They attract moisture from the atmosphere and the epidermis and bind water to the skin. Moisturizers temporarily replenish the skin and smooth fine lines and wrinkles found in most moisturizers. They are especially beneficial for oilier, dehydrated skin. Humectants include hexanediol, butylene glycol, glycerin, and sorbitol, while hyaluronic acid is also used as a humectant.

- **Occlusives**

These moisturizers coat the outermost layer of the epidermis, the stratum corneum, and prevent transepidermal water loss (TEWL). They are less cosmetically desirable and are generally recommended on a professional basis for people suffering from psoriasis, eczema, and other skin conditions. Common occlusives may include cocoa butter, shea butter, propylene glycol and beeswax.

Eye Products

The skin around the eyes is very delicate and needs special care, at least good care if you are not looking for something extraordinary. The skin around the eyes is thin and fragile, and a product that is good for facial skin is usually good for the eyes as well, unless the products are not used to combat oily skin or treat a specific skin condition.

There are two camps when we talk about eye products:

- Those who really enjoy using it and want to see the benefits.

- And those who think it is unnecessary and a waste of money.

Before making a decision for or against the use of eye contour products, be very clear that everything that happens around you affects the eye area and that the health of all your internal organs is clearly reflected in them.

Eye contour products often contain ingredients such as green tea, caffeine, and peptides to combat dark circles, bags, and wrinkles. No eye contour product is a permanent "remedy": all ethical brands advise constant use, as the effect of a product disappears if you stop using it.

<u>Things to Do and Avoid</u>

- Using mineral oils around your eye area tends to make the area puffy. Only the lightest of serums can be used on the eyelids.

- Usage of more than the advised amount of cream could cause irritation and – waste of money, of course.

- Thicker creams on the lids are good for eczema or psoriasis in the eye area – that may be prescribed by your doctor depending on the severity of your condition.

- Keep it simple – fragrant eye products can really irritate the eye area.

- The ingredient, bismuth oxychloride, causes most allergies to eye products and eyeshadows/mineral makeup, which is used to give the shimmery' glow.' If your mineral makeup makes you itch, check their INCI list to spot out bismuth oxychloride.

Exfoliation

Exfoliation is an essential step in a good skincare routine that should be performed fairly frequently. Exfoliation removes dirt and dead skin cells that have accumulated on the top layer of skin, resulting in an uneven and dull skin tone. Exfoliating regularly improves skin texture, removes blackheads, and allows serum and moisturizer to penetrate effectively.

There are two methods of exfoliation.

- **Mechanical exfoliators**

These exfoliants include sponges, scrubs, facial brushes, and electronic cleansing devices. Scrubs with sugar, crystals, or other rough particles help to effectively remove dead skin cells, reduce blackheads and unclog pores. In comparison, exfoliation devices can effectively clean hard-to-reach areas, such as the sides of the nose, but they can be harsh and damage the skin.

- **Chemical exfoliators**

For this type of exfoliation you cannot do it yourself, but have to go to a suitable professional. Exfoliating acids are used to remove dead cells and dirt from the face, without any pain. Acids make the skin smoother and brighter. Pick up exfoliants containing alpha-hydroxy acids (AHAs), beta hydroxy acids (BHAs), and polyhydroxy acids, depending on your skin's needs. Chemical exfoliants are recommended for the following cases:

1. If your skin is showing signs of aging.

2. If you suffer from blemishes, spots, or acne.

3. If you want the beneficial effects of acid for sensitive and problematic skin.

Exfoliation methods, frequency, and products for exfoliation depend solely on the type and condition of your skin. Oily skin can tolerate daily or every other day exfoliation, while weekly exfoliation may be more than sufficient for dry or sensitive skin. Excessive exfoliation, even on oily and acne-prone skin, can remove the lipid layer and leave the skin more inflamed and sore.

Face Masks

Face masks are a luxurious way to spend some downtime, but they clearly don't provide any long-term benefits to the skin. However, sheet masks are a better way to invest time in yourself for a positive impact on mental health, wellness, and stress reduction.

- Masks with clay, charcoal, salicylic acid, glycolic acid, witch hazel, niacinamide, and tea tree oil, to name a few, are beneficial for oily skin types.

- Sheet masks or masks infused with hyaluronic acid are generally good for dry or dehydrated skin that needs a radiance boost.

- Brightening masks with vitamin C can help liven up the dull skin.

Face masks have a positive impact on the skin during long-term air travel and others. There is nothing wrong with using face masks regularly, unless they suit your skin type without any irritation, redness, flaking, or sensitivity. We'll see more about face masks in the next chapter.

Sunscreen

There is certainly no difference of opinion on the use of sunscreen as an essential element in the daily skincare regimen. Sunscreen protects the skin against solar radiation.

Daily use of a sunscreen is strongly advised, and yes, one should not stop using it during the cloudy season, but regular use throughout the year is a must. Especially for people who spend a good deal of time outdoors in the sun or who regularly exfoliate their skin with AHAs and BHAs, regular use of sunscreens becomes a must.

Sunscreens are available in different formulations. Those with dry skin should use a balm or cream-rich sunscreen. For oily skin, a fluid texture or a light gel with a matte finish is recommended. People with sensitive skin should use sunscreens containing titanium dioxide and zinc oxide.

Sunscreens are usually moisturizers, and for people with oily skin, it is not necessary to apply moisturizer before sunscreen; it may be sufficient on its own.

Half a teaspoon of sunscreen is considered a good amount to apply to the face and neck.

CHAPTER 7:

Your Skin: Facial Masks

A facial mask is a temporary covering applied to the surface of the skin, usually to moisturize, protect against external irritants or exfoliate. Facial masks are usually applied once or twice a week, before bedtime, to give the user time to sleep while the mask minimizes signs of aging.

Facial masks can be simple or complex. Complex masks are usually made by a pharmacist and require a doctor's prescription. These masks use synthetic mixtures of chemical compounds that have been carefully formulated to treat specific skin conditions.

In addition to masking the effects of aging, facial masks can also provide several health benefits by reducing inflammation and relieving stress.

Types of Facial Mask

There are many types of facial masks. Some examples are listed below. It is important to keep in mind that these are very generalized classifications and there is often overlap between them.

Choosing the right face mask depends on several factors, such as skin type, available ingredients, budget, etc. Many people try several before finding one that works for their skin.

Clay Mask

This mask uses clay because it has a high absorption capacity and acts like a magnet, drawing out impurities and dead skin cells that can clog pores and cause acne breakouts and blackheads.

Application example.

To make a paste, combine one tablespoon of powdered clay (French green clay is my favorite) with two tablespoons of water or apple cider vinegar. Apply it in circular motions to the face, avoiding the eye area.

Sheet Mask

If you're going out, a face mask is a perfect way to refresh your face quickly. Sheet masks are made of paper soaked in a moisturizing or anti-aging formula or serum.

Application: After cleansing your face, open the container and take out the sheet mask. Apply the mask evenly over the face. Avoid the eye area. Let it sit for about 15-18 minutes before removing it and apply the excess essence to your skin.

Cream Mask

Cream masks are easy to apply and are not usually messy. Cream masks are used to moisturize the skin.

Application: Apply a thin layer of the cream mask to your face, avoiding the eye area, leaving it on for 10-15 minutes before removing it with water.

Oil Mask

Oil masks are usually best for those with oily skin. Oil masks are very popular because they leave the skin very lightly scented and moisturized.

Application: After cleansing your face, apply a drop or two of your favorite oil (olive oil is my favorite) to your face and let it absorb into your skin for 10 minutes before removing and patting the excess essence into your skin.

Gel Mask

Gel masks are a good alternative to cream and oil. They are suitable for all skin types, even sensitive skin.

Application: After cleansing your face, apply a small amount of gel mask to your face and leave it on for 15-18 minutes before removing it and patting the excess essence into your skin.

Charcoal Masks

Charcoal mask is a very popular type of face mask. It is activated charcoal that helps to draw out excess oil from the pores.

Examples of charcoal face masks

- **Activated Charcoal Mask -** This mask purifies the pores while absorbing all the dirt and pollution. It has a good cooling effect on your skin to soothe irritated problems.

- **The Green Tea Mask -** This mask contains actual pieces of green tea leaves for drinkability sake. You can apply it generously and leave it on for up to 10 minutes to get any benefit from the amino acids in green tea.

Application Tips

Mix a small amount of coconut oil and a little water to form a paste, then mix the activated charcoal to form a thick paste. Apply it on the face with circular movements. Leave it on for about 20 minutes before removing it and washing it off with lukewarm water.

Peel-Off Mask

Peel-off masks use the power of permanent adhesives to adhere to one side of the skin and then peel off like a sticker. The benefits are pretty obvious: they provide great coverage, are durable enough to wear daily, and can be removed at any time. But there's one important thing to consider before buying one: what type of skin you have. There are many peel-off masks tailored to different skin types, which could increase their effectiveness or even prevent any problems that might arise with specific types.

Application: Apply a thin layer evenly all over the face. Wait about 10 minutes before removing slowly.

CHAPTER 8:

Your Skin: Benefits Of Body Scrubs

This chapter introduces you to the benefits of body scrub for your skin. It also contains some tips to help you choose the best body scrub for your skin type. It is well known that when we take care of our skin, it in turn takes care of us. Therefore, it is important to choose a product that takes care of our skin's needs and concerns. One way to make sure the skin is happy is to use a body scrub at least once or twice a week.

A body scrub not only cleanses the top layer of dead cells, but also stimulates cell turnover, which causes an increase in collagen production, thus improving elasticity and reducing age spots, wrinkles, stretch marks, etc. The large amount of vitamin A contained in the scrub promotes cell renewal and regeneration, making the skin glow. The unique blend of ingredients used in the product will also help improve skin texture. It is important to select a scrub that contains an adequate amount of lubricant to prevent redness, irritation, and dryness. Your choice should contain natural ingredients such as chamomile, lemon juice, rose petals, and essential oils such as extracts of geranium, lavender, or marshmallow root. In addition, you should choose a scrub formulated with gentle clays such as kaolin or bentonite clay, which have been shown to help reduce fine lines and wrinkles. If you're not blessed with the smooth, clear complexion of a teenager or someone who has never worn makeup or used sunscreen, you'll want to select an exfoliant that contains keratin to slow the aging process. This is because keratin helps repair damaged skin and encourages cell growth, which makes the skin look younger and healthier. Combining all this with gentle exfoliation can make your skin glow and give it a healthy glow. Body scrubs are not only an effective way to exfoliate and moisturize the skin, but can also be used as a facial mask to benefit your complexion.

Body Scrubs Tips

Use a body scrub 3 to 4 times a month to give your skin the deep exfoliation it needs. Before showering, pat your skin dry with a towel and massage the scrub over all areas of your body, following the instructions on the bottle. You can also use it on your feet or elbows before going to bed. Avoid sensitive areas such as the face, chest, and genitals. Rinse with lukewarm water before entering the shower to prevent the product from building up and clogging pores (especially important for people with sensitive skin). Next, apply a body lotion or cream to lock in moisture.

You can find a variety of exfoliating body scrubs in drugstores and most department stores; most contain the same basic ingredients.

Examples of Body Scrubs

Examples of Body scrub products you can buy from stores are:

- Bath and Body Works Coconut Lime Verbena Shea Butter Marshmallow Hand Soap, 12 Fl oz (Pack of 4)

- Essential Rosemary Mint Handmade Soap

- Aveeno Skin Relief Body Wash with Natural Oat Extract & Shea Butter for Dry, Irritated Skin - 24 Fl. Oz. - Pack of 2

- LUSH Cosmetics First Aid Beauty Cream 8oz

These are just examples, you can choose the exfoliator that suits you best. Choose products that have the smallest possible grain size, as this allows for better exfoliation. You can also add your own natural ingredients from home. Homemade scrubs work just as well, with the added bonus of being all-natural for anyone who cares about what goes on their skin.

Here are the examples of home-made body scrubs you can try at home:

- **Olive oil and sugar:** This is a tried-and-true combination that gives your skin exfoliation and easy hydration. Scrub gently on damp skin with a mixture of one-part olive oil and three parts sugar to eliminate dead cells from the epidermis' outer layer. After five minutes, rinse with warm water.

- **Salt, sugar, and lemon juice:** Mix two tablespoons of salt with two tablespoons of organic cane sugar. Add a tablespoon of fresh lemon juice and work into a paste in your hands. Spread over your body and gently scrub away. Rinse off with water after five minutes.

- **Baking soda:** Mix 6 teaspoons of baking soda with distilled water and gently massage into the skin. Rinse off with water after five minutes to remove any remaining baking soda residue.

- **Vitamin E:** This is a gentle oil on the skin that penetrates deeply and moisturizes dry skin. Pat onto the entire body -- especially on elbows, knees, and heels -- and allow to absorb for five minutes. Rinse off with warm water after. Vitamin E also improves skin elasticity and reduces wrinkles by stimulating collagen production in the dermis (the layers of the epidermis below the outer layer of dead cells). It also protects against UV damage, which may help prevent premature signs of aging.

- **Neem oil:** This is an extreme-rating oil, so be careful when using it. Its antimicrobial properties help to kill bacteria, which includes what causes acne and acne scars. It reaches directly to the roots of these issues, so it should be used with care since it may cause irritation. Neem has been shown to affect the production of hormones that stimulate the growth of hair follicles by starving the cells that build viruses that cause acne. This oil helps prevent any bacteria from growing further. The best way to use neem oil is by mixing it with water (to dilute the active ingredient) and applying it like body wash. Neem can be used on all parts of the body, except for anal areas, where you might have irritation after using this product. Use this oil two times a day, once in the morning and once before bed.

- **Tea tree oil:** This is an essential oil that comes from the Melaleuca alternifolia plant in Australia. It has antimicrobial properties to prevent the growth of bacteria (which includes acne). You can find tea tree oil in lotions, creams, and many other natural products. To make a paste, combine 1 tablespoon powder clay with 2 tablespoons of water or apple cider vinegar. Apply to your face in circular motions. Avoid applying on the eye area.

- **Mango butter:** This is a useful treatment for dry skin. The texture is similar to that of sebum oil; it penetrates deep into the dermis and moisturizes the skin. It's a terrific option for persons with sensitive skin because mango butter is relatively mild compared to other nut butters and won't irritate them.

Making Your Own Customized Homemade Body Scrub Recipe

By following these steps, you can make your own body scrub at home with your favorite ingredients. If the above DIY scrubs are not to your liking, you can try this one.

- 1/2 cup oil (for example, shea butter, coconut oil, olive oil)

- 1/4 cup sugar (for example, cane sugar, brown sugar)

- 1 teaspoon salt (Kosher or sea salt work well, but some people prefer Himalayan pink salt)

- 12-15 drops essential oils (optional, but I recommend some citrus oils like lemon or orange to brighten up your scrub)

- Pour all the ingredients into a bowl

Your scrub is ready to use.

CHAPTER 9:

Your Skin: Common Skin Problems

The condition of our skin is something that fluctuates throughout our lifetime and is affected by several factors:

- Diet

- Lifestyle

- Weather

- Where we live – e.g., coastal or town location

- Pollution

- Age

- Sun exposure

Here are the Common Skin Conditions and Solutions:

Dehydration

You get dehydration when you have low water content in the skin.

Solution

1. Always use a toner. This is a step often left out of the skincare regime, but regular use will improve hydration levels.

2. Exfoliate. A build-up of dead skin cells will form a barrier to the active ingredients in skincare products.

3. Check your environment. Workplaces with central heating or air conditioning can dehydrate the skin.

4. Drink more water. This can be in the form of decaffeinated teas as well as water, but preferably excluding sugar content. Drinking water during exercise is beneficial, too, since it transfers to other areas of the body and can nourish the skin within a short space of time.

Skin Dulling

Dull skin is recognized as a distinct lack of color, where the appearance of the skin is pale as a result of a lack of circulation in the upper layers of the skin. This is often seen in long-term smokers as a result of poor circulation and free radical damage to the surface of the skin.

Oily skin can sometimes be dull and lack color, due to a thicker epidermis, in addition to the reasons mentioned above. After many years of sun exposure, mature skin may have a thicker epidermis, an accumulation of dead skin cells, and a dull appearance.

Solution

Exfoliating will help with dullness to some extent, but it is important to create a balance between exfoliation and stimulating circulation. Spirulina is a great example of a stimulating ingredient. By stimulating circulation, color, and oxygen rise to the surface of the skin. It can be used after an exfoliating product or equally on its own. Use a mask with spirulina to stimulate circulation, giving the skin a translucent and radiant appearance.

Massage stimulates skin circulation, increases color by boosting blood flow to the skin's surface, and improves suppleness and absorption of oils: an easy home care option for dull skin.

Wrinkles and Fine Lines

Fine lines and wrinkles can be evidence of dehydration and the first signs of aging.

Solution

1. Protect the skin with an SPF (minimum factor 30) during the summer. Winter protection can be provided in your foundation (if you wear one) or an SPF moisturizer (factor 15–25, if you spend more time outdoors than most people).

2. The sun damages collagen and elastin and will lead to sagging, fine lines, and/or wrinkles as a result of the breakdown of the skin's fibrous structures.

3. Use a vitamin C skincare product to stimulate collagen and elastin production. The percentage of vitamin C can vary, but I recommend you start at 3-5%, gradually increasing to 15- 20% as your skin adapts. The higher levels are not suitable for sensitive skins, so I would always start a lower level first and build up to the higher levels if your skin responds positively.

4. Increase vitamin C in your diet. This is the body's main nutrient source for collagen and elastin. If you're experiencing stress, then an increase in the intake of vitamin C – and all antioxidants – is recommended to combat free radicals.

5. Topical applications help to slow the aging process by neutralizing free radicals and offering protection from UV rays.

6. You can hydrate superficial fine lines using toners, serums, and masques. And increase moisture levels using face oils and creams.

7. A high sugar intake is commonly believed to exacerbate this condition, so moderating sugar levels is a great idea.

8. Use products rich in antioxidants to combat free radical damage. This is a great opportunity to use natural-based serums, masques, and moisturizers.

Pigmentation

Pigmentation is usually caused by overexposure to the sun. When we tan, the skin produces melanin, which gives it a golden brown appearance. Repeated exposure to the sun alters melanin production, so that the skin continues to produce melanin whether or not it is exposed to the sun. The most common signs of this are unconventional brown marks and spots on the skin. While the rest of the skin returns to its normal color when the tan fades, the brown marks remain, darkening each time they are exposed to the sun.

Protection against sun damage:

Use (at a minimum) SPF 30 when your skin is exposed to the sun for prolonged periods. This is not a guarantee against pigmentation, but it will help minimize and delay any visible signs of sun damage. Check in your regular skincare to see if an extra high SPF factor is necessary.

Facial hair removal can make the treated area more susceptible to pigmentation.

Products that lighten or reduce pigmentation come in different forms. It is easier to lighten skin, but ending established pigmentation is more difficult.

Any sun exposure will stimulate melanin production, even when a high sun protection factor has been applied. Prevention is better than any cure.

There is no quick fix or definitive cure for this condition. Everyone's case is different, so understanding your skin triggers is a very important factor in managing this condition.

Common Triggers:

1. Spicy food

2. Red wine

3. Extreme hot/cold weather

4. Stress

5. Hormonal changes

6. A climate change – going on holiday, or to or moving to a new environment, where weather, pollution levels, water, and Lifestyle are radically different.

Your skin condition can be treated with an effective daily skincare regimen, with the addition of serums chosen specifically for your symptoms. It can be difficult to find the right products for your personalized skincare regimen. Always test products before committing to long-term use and look for formulas designed for rosacea and not for all skin types.

Sensitive Skin

Most of us are not born with sensitivity, but some skin types are more susceptible. Sensitivity can be caused by any of the following factors:

- A weaker/thin epidermis is found in dry skin types. Extreme weather conditions can accelerate this condition.

- Certain harsh products can cause sensitivity in any skin type by disrupting the skin's barrier (acid mantle).

- Products containing raw, organic, or unrefined ingredients can cause sensitivity due to their active properties.

- Extreme hot or cold weather can cause sensitivity, either from sunburn or low temperatures.

- Regular use of acid peels followed by sun exposure may accelerate or cause sensitivity.

You can add the above conditions that concern you most in order of priority. This will form an important tool for guiding your choice of products.

CHAPTER 10:

Your Skin: Dealing With Acne

Millions of people suffer embarrassment and discouragement because of acne. Most are found in adolescence, but adults are also affected. There are numerous acne treatment options on the market, some of which are well formulated while others are less effective. Finding the best acne skin treatments can help you feel better about yourself and your appearance.

Acne Treatment Tips

Natural and gentle products are the best choices for acne treatment. Look for botanical ingredients in the ingredient list. Sage, yarrow, horsenail, wild thyme, horsetail, milkweed, and peppermint are some of the herbal ingredients that help heal blemished skin. Aloe vera is a known skin healer that is often ineffective in acne treatments. Some essential oils can also help in the treatment of acne. Some essential oils are irritating to the skin. (The best acne treatment products may contain oils such as lavender, rose, tangerine, and geranium. These are not only beneficial to the skin, but also enhance the scent of the product.

If the product is designed with a transdermal system, the vitamins or herbal ingredients will absorb into the skin and treat the acne at its source. Vitamin C, A, E, and provitamin B5 are some of the vitamins that can be included in topical acne treatment.

The best acne treatment, like healthy foods for the body, will provide nutrients and nourishment directly to the skin. The skin often reveals a person's health. What appears on the outside usually indicates an internal deficiency or need. Eating a healthy diet can help overcome acne and is a good complement to using good products.

However, even the best products will not eliminate acne if used inconsistently. It is a good idea to establish a daily routine of taking vitamin supplements and cleansing your face. Don't let procrastination or disorganization deprive you of time to take care of yourself. The skin is the largest organ of the body and plays an important role in eliminating toxins from the body. It requires pampering and care. Moisturizer is also an essential component of acne treatment. Like the other components, it must be completely natural, otherwise, it will clog pores and worsen the situation. Read the label carefully to make sure the ingredients are all-natural botanicals, nutrients, and healthy oils.

Some people recommend that you only use products on your skin that you would put in your mouth. This is not always the case because the skin acts as a filter when absorbing nutrients and other substances. On the other hand, the use of unnatural products should be avoided.

Simple Health That Would Prevent You from Getting Acne

Drink Plenty of Water

Water has long been considered the most effective or almost free natural treatment for any skin condition because of its alkaline pH of 7.3. It prevents dehydration, which allows the sebaceous glands to produce sebum or oil. The skin needs water to function properly, so doctors and nutritionists recommend drinking 6 to 8 glasses of water a day.

Proper Diet

Skin health is also influenced by nutrition. Some foods are said to cause allergic reactions in some people. Chocolate is currently a hotly debated topic in the field of nutrition. Some say chocolate improves skin condition, while others say it does not. Whatever the case, the best advice is to eat a healthy diet high in fiber and fresh fruits and vegetables.

A Healthy Facial Care Routine

When it comes to facial skincare, establishing a healthy beauty routine is beneficial. Most doctors today advise cleansing, moisturizing, and toning the skin twice a day. When cleansing, never forget to cleanse the neck area, including the face. Then apply a moisturizer or neck cream.

Avoid Overexposure to the Sun

Sunburn is caused by overexposure to sunlight, as you may already know. So even though today's sunscreens only block UVB rays while allowing harmful UVA rays in, it's still wise to cover up before getting into Apollo's hands. To keep the sun off your face while gardening, wear a wide-brimmed hat.

Exercise

In addition to eating a healthy diet, exercising your body also contributes to skin health. It is important to keep in mind that proper exercise not only keeps the body in shape by regulating oxygen levels, but it also improves the glow of the skin.

Get Enough Rest

When stressed, the adrenal cortex converts adrenal androgens into the hormone testosterone, which causes hyperactivity of the sebaceous glands in both men and women. Due to dehydration, these adrenal androgens cause a double amount of testosterone to be produced, which causes the face to become greasy.

CHAPTER 11:

Your Teeth:
Whitening And Maintenance

We all know the basics of oral care, from brushing and flossing to relieving toothaches and fighting cavities.

In this and the following chapters, we are going to focus on tooth care topics that impact our beauty, such as teeth whitening, protective maintenance, interdental cleaning, and the importance of dental visits.

We always set out to whiten our teeth. And at the same time, we would like to avoid having teeth stains and other dental problems.

Take a look at what you should avoid doing to keep those teeth stains from happening to your teeth. And a few simple reminders on what you should do every day to keep your teeth white for a long, long time.

Brushing

Brushing is the most common oral health technique. Dentists usually recommend brushing at least twice a day or, preferably, at every meal. When brushing your teeth, remember not to rush. Oral health experts say to brush your teeth for at least two minutes.

Here's the simple way to brush your teeth.

- Start with the outer part of your upper teeth. Brush your teeth using a circular motion.

- Do the same for the outer part of your lower teeth.

- After that, brush the part of the teeth that you use for chewing.

To have a fresher breath, dentists advise that you also brush your tongue.

The type of toothbrush is also important. People with sensitive gums will have difficulty brushing their teeth comfortably if they use a toothbrush with hard bristles. Toothbrushes with small bristles are recommended to avoid damaging the gums. Small-headed brushes are better because they can reach the innermost parts of our mouth. The choice of the handle will depend on your comfort: there are no rules.

There are two types of toothbrushes on the market today: manual and electric. The choice will depend on the situation and your preferences. If dexterity is your problem, you can opt for an electric toothbrush.

Brushing Too Much and Too Less Are Not Advisable

We have to brush our teeth every day. That is a must. What we should not do is to brush our teeth too much. We should not brush more than necessary.

How many times should you brush your teeth? Dentists recommend at least twice a day. You should brush once in the morning and before going to bed at night.

Some people brush after every time they put food in their mouth. Others brush for no reason and out of habit many times during the day. You should not brush excessively, or your tooth enamel will thin. As you know, enamel protects your teeth from decay and gives them their normal color.

The ability of your tooth enamel to tolerate or delay thinning decreases as we age. Brushing your teeth too hard accelerates enamel thinning as you age.

If you should avoid over-brushing, you should also avoid under-brushing. Not brushing your teeth when you need to is inviting bacteria from the outside (especially from the food you eat) to build up.

Bacteria in the mouth create dental plaque in just two days of not brushing. And, in just ten days, that plaque turns into tartar, which is worse. Don't forget to brush your teeth every day.

Brushing your teeth removes food particles that turn into bacteria. Plaque is that yellow gunk that makes your teeth yellow. If you don't brush your teeth or don't brush at all, your teeth are sure to become discolored.

Avoid Biting Too Hard

You should not bite too hard with your teeth. When eating foods that are difficult to chew, do not force yourself to bite down hard to chew them.

Cut food into smaller pieces with the appropriate tool: a dining room knife or kitchen knife. You do not need to use your teeth to cut food.

Don't use your teeth like a pair of scissors or a sharp knife. If you do this as if you were tearing the skin off sugar cane, you are exposing your teeth to breaking and bleeding. You can also accidentally bite your tongue, and that is extremely painful.

Avoid using your teeth to open a bottle cap, which others do to show off their strong teeth. Cracking nuts with your teeth is another forbidden method.

Grinding Teeth

If you now grind your teeth for a medical reason such as when you are nervous or anxious, you should see a doctor for an examination. You should avoid grinding your teeth, as it can also lead to the darkening of the teeth.

Bruxism is a disorder that causes people to grind their teeth while sleeping. If you notice that you have this disorder, get it checked out right away.

In a physical activity such as doing heavy manual labor or playing sports that make you concentrate intensely, you may be grinding your teeth and not be aware of it. It is similar to bruxism, and you should find out how you can avoid it. Also, avoid injuring your face from too much physical activity. Getting hit in the face would mean getting hit in the teeth or jolted.

Stay Away from Chemicals

Avoid eating or drinking anything bad for your teeth. There are some chemicals in them that are bad for your teeth. These chemicals make your teeth stained.

You should cut down or avoid drinking red wine, tea, cola, and coffee. Too much of these liquids can cause your teeth to stain. When stains appear on your teeth, the enamel will wear away. You will have worse problems than just stains on your teeth.

Even natural foods like apples, potatoes, and rice can cause discoloration of your teeth. Carbohydrates have a sugar content that plaque feeds on. When this happens, the enamel has no way to prevent bacteria from settling in if there are too many carbohydrates left on your teeth.

Fluorosis is an excess of fluoride that can cause teeth to turn brown. Fluoride is not only used in toothpaste. It is also a component of bottled fruit drinks or processed juices. Avoid drinking these fluoridated beverages.

Using Mouthwash & Medicines

Mouthwash is good when you like to rinse after brushing your teeth. You should know that some mouthwashes have essential oils that are bad for your teeth. These oils are meant to scent your mouth, but these oils can cause stains on your teeth. You should reduce or avoid using mouthwashes.

Antibiotics and other medications containing tetracycline, minocycline, and ciprofloxacin can cause stains on your teeth with strange colors such as green, gray, blue, brown, and bright yellow.

Teeth Whitening Methods

Conventional Whitening Methods

Conventional methods include bleaching, dental masks, and whitening toothpaste. These methods are effective with some disadvantages.

The dentist can make your teeth white with whitening procedures. However, these are expensive and are only temporary. Even teeth whitening kits that have a lower price tag may even make your situation worse. Dental veneers don't help either because the integrity of the teeth is sacrificed when the dentist scrapes away the enamel to make way for the veneers and resins to adhere to the teeth.

Even whitening toothpaste doesn't guarantee anything at all. You may be buying a whitening toothpaste that doesn't work anyway and is more expensive than regular toothpaste.

Home Remedies for Whitening

On the other side of the medicine, there is the unconventional method. This is commonly known as a home remedy. This category for teeth whitening is further classified into long-term effects, short-term effects, and herbal medicine.

You should first evaluate what type of teeth whitening home remedy is appropriate for you to make sure you don't run into problems later on.

Here are some of the recommended long-term home remedies:

- **Pure baking soda** - free radicals from the water-dissolved baking soda penetrate the teeth' enamel to lighten the stain of brown or yellow to a much whiter appearance.

- **Baking soda and toothpaste** - both baking soda and toothpaste have the ingredients of cleaning the enamel.

- **Baking soda and glycerin** - these two together as a thicker paste and can be effective to whiten a discolored tooth because it has the qualities of whitening paste.

- **Olive oil and diluted apple cider** - when mixed, is said to clean and whiten teeth because of the abrasive and acidic properties that rub off the stain off the discolored teeth.

- **Hydrogen peroxide** - works as a mouth rinse. After mixing it with water, it becomes a powerful rinse that dislodges all debris on the teeth.

Here are some of the short-term home-based remedies:

- Pure lemon juice

- Lemon juice and rock salt

- Pure hardwood ash

- Hardwood ash and toothpaste

- Vinegar and baking soda.

There are also traditional home remedies that use natural ingredients such as orange peels, basal leaves, crushed walnuts, green walnut shells, a mixture of turmeric powder, salt and mustard oil, sesame seeds, and many more. However, you may not find them easily.

Online resources, including YouTube, are readily available on how to perform these teeth whitening methods.

Keep in mind that home remedies for teeth whitening are not commonly used, and their effectiveness also depends on the correct procedure for making the mixture or compound.

Remember also that home remedies are not recommended for children under 17 years of age. Dental fillings, veneers, braces, orthodontic appliances, and other similar structures may also be affected. It is strongly recommended not to use home remedies if you have cracks in your teeth, gum damage, and other dental defects. Dental fillings, veneers, braces and other similar tooth structures done by the dentist will be affected by home remedies, so better watch out for them.

It would be best to consult a dentist before doing any teeth whitening program. A dentist is still best suited to determine if your tooth enamel is robust enough to tolerate abrasive and acidic whitening treatments. However, if the dentist has certified that your teeth have strong enamel and will be able to protect them by making a home remedy for teeth whitening, thank him or her and make the remedy yourself. If you have tried a home remedy, wait a while to see the effects before trying another remedy. Preferably, if a remedy has already worked, stick with it.

CHAPTER 12:

Your Teeth:
The Practice Of Interdental Cleaning

D
o you know what is the most vulnerable area of the mouth, prone to periodontal disease and tooth decay? It is the space between two teeth (interdental space), which cannot be adequately cleaned with the help of a normal toothbrush. It is also the most neglected area, even if a rigid oral hygiene regimen is followed. Despite meticulous attempts to maintain oral hygiene to the utmost, tooth sensitivity, tooth decay, and inflamed gums manifest. To further halt the progression of the disease, interdental cleaning becomes essential.

What is Interdental Cleaning?

Cleaning the space between two adjacent teeth is called interdental cleaning. It is crucial, otherwise, all efforts to maintain optimal oral health are in vain. Brushing and interdental cleaning, twice a day, saves costly dental visits and treatments, as well as precious time. It is a fact that dirty interdental spaces are a breeding ground for bacteria, leading to the onset and progression of periodontal disease and dental caries.

Unhygienic interdental spaces give rise to undesirable consequences like:

- Interdental Teeth Cavities

- Sensitivity

- Gum and Periodontal Infections

- Bad Breath

Putrification of the food entrapped in the interdental spaces causes offensive breath.

Interdental Cleaning Tools

Interdental cleaning is essential for maintaining oral and general health. Several interdental cleaning aids have been designed and are available on the market.

Toothpicks

By far the most convenient interdental cleaning utensil. Toothpicks are made of wood or plastic, with one or both pointed ends, for insertion between the teeth. Toothpicks are used to push food material stuck between the teeth. Toothpicks are excellent tools for cleaning slightly open interdental areas and should be used with caution.

Interdental Brushes

They are classified into two types. The Uni-tuft brush and the miniature bottle cleaning brush.

The Uni-tuft brush is used in the open contact areas, to dislodge food particles, while the miniature bottle cleaning brush is used to maintain and clean the interdental areas of recessed gums.

Dental Floss

Simple floss is a piece of thin, clean floss. It passes and slides between the teeth, when held between the index fingers of both hands and pushed along the space between the two adjacent teeth. Then, with a slight movement of both hands, the floss is gently moved back and forth to clean the interdental space.

Floss Picker

Another type of prepared flosser is a combination flosser and toothpick. It has a plastic handle with a pointed end (the pick end), while the other end holds the floss in a side-facing U shape. It is used with one hand.

An Oral Irrigator

This is the ultimate interdental cleaning aid with several advantages. This device holds a tip attached to a water reservoir. Pulsed jets of pressurized water, generated by a built-in pump, enter the tip of the irrigator. The tip is directed into the interdental spaces. This dislodges plaque and food. The irrigator is suitable for sensitive gums and teeth. It mechanically stimulates the gingiva, improving blood flow and thus gingival health.

The main purpose of interdental cleaning is to remove food debris and plaque. The bristles of a toothbrush cannot penetrate the narrow interdental spaces, so interdental cleaning devices are very useful. To ensure optimal cleaning of the interdental region and to maintain good oral hygiene, the use of the above-mentioned devices is necessary.

CHAPTER 13:

Your Teeth: More Dental Health Tips

In general, it is recommended to visit the dentist for a periodic check-up at least once every six months, if not sooner if personal needs dictate. It is better to visit a dentist to rule out the possibility of a dental and oral ailment than to wait until it is symptomatic. By the time most dental ailments become symptomatic, they have already begun to reach an irreversible stage.

Preservation is the Key

As we know, there is no artificial substitute that can replace the natural one. The majority professional opinion is that the natural tooth structure should be preserved as much as possible. Therefore, it would be unwise to remove existing teeth that can be saved to make a prosthesis. Dentures have their own problems and limitations. Full dentures are believed to carry, at best, one-sixth to one-fifth of the load that natural teeth carry. Dentures may force you to significantly alter what and how you eat. This can impact your eating habits and, in some cases, your nutrition. The link between choking and denture wear also seems strong. And choking on food seems to be a fairly common cause of accidental death. Dentures need regular maintenance and must be replaced or repaired every few years. In addition, dentures are expensive. Natural teeth are free, more effective, and last much longer with little attention and care. Please discuss in detail with your dentist before jumping into the decision to extract teeth for dentures. Modern dentistry offers not only excellent treatment options, but very effective preventive strategies to rid you of your dental ailments. You can also save yourself the time and cost of maintenance, provided you develop a meticulous oral prophylaxis routine.

Toothbrush Versus Toothpaste

Without a doubt, the toothbrush is more important than toothpaste. In fact, it is a properly selected and maintained toothbrush used with proper brushing technique that is very important. However, a good toothpaste can help when used in conjunction with a good toothbrush and proper brushing technique. One of the most effective tools in preventive dentistry is the use of fluoride toothpaste. This toothpaste contains about 400 to 1000 parts per million of fluoride and is considered very effective in remineralizing teeth and preventing tooth decay.

Prevention of Dental Caries

Many diseases of the teeth and gums can be totally prevented if our mouth is kept absolutely clean. Keeping the mouth clean means effectively cleaning and removing the layer of plaque that accumulates on the teeth and adjacent gums. It is not possible to have a 24-hour plaque-free mouth, as plaque begins to form almost immediately after teeth cleaning. However, most experts believe that meticulous plaque removal at least once a day, using all necessary oral prophylactic means, is sufficient to prevent caries and gum disease.

Removing Plaque from Teeth

The basic armamentarium to effectively remove plaque and delay its reformation consists of a proper toothbrush used with the appropriate brushing technique, adequate floss for interdental cleaning, and an appropriate mouth rinse. The efficacy of plaque removal can be evaluated and improved by intermittent use of a plaque disclosing agent.

In addition to following these methods of oral prophylaxis, proper dietary modification, including content and timing (avoiding intermediate or frequent snacking), and gargling after each food intake will help improve oral hygiene. Regular visits to the dental office and cleaning (scaling) of the teeth in the office will help maintain clean teeth and a healthy oral cavity.

Over time, plaque may calcify and tartar deposits may develop on the teeth. Also, the teeth may develop extrinsic stains. These stains and tartar are impossible for the patient to remove with standard teeth cleaning methods and require the dentist to use special equipment and instruments to remove them from the teeth. The purpose of scaling is to remove these external stains and tartar from the surface of the teeth and to smooth the exposed tooth roots so that the patient can effectively clean them of plaque with regular teeth cleaning methods. Proper and meticulous scaling of the teeth is harmless, if not beneficial.

After scaling the teeth, patients usually experience slight tooth sensitivity, occasionally increased tooth mobility, and the perception of increased space between teeth. These are incidental and usually temporary findings and should not be perceived as the detrimental effects of scaling. In fact, scaling has revealed the deleterious effects of calculus and ineffective maintenance of oral hygiene. Bleeding that may occur during the scaling process also stops immediately after scaling and should not cause much concern.

Benefits of Dental Floss

Dental floss is a floss used to clean interdental surfaces. Proper brushing of the teeth helps reduce plaque on most areas of the teeth. However, the areas of the teeth below and above their proximal contact points remain inaccessible to the bristles of the toothbrush. These are the areas where flossing helps. Dental floss can come in several varieties. They can be single or multifilament. They can be waxed or unwaxed. They can be continuous or segmented. Each type of floss has its own indications for use. Most people recommend a flat, waxed, continuous, multifilament floss for regular flossing. To clean the undersurfaces of a fixed bridge, a segmented floss can be used. If you have never heard of dental floss, you may be tempted to think that it is something very new for oral hygiene.

Other Dental Tools

Most of us are familiar with a toothbrush and toothpaste to clean our teeth. However, some other tools and devices can be used to clean teeth from plaque and food debris. Among them, the most commonly used are dental floss, interdental brushes, special wooden tips for interdental cleaning, oral irrigation tips and devices, various medicated and non-medicated mouth rinses, disclosing solutions, and, most importantly, lots of motivation!

Smoking and Your Dental Health

The widespread harmful effects of smoking are well documented. However, local effects due to tobacco chewing can further aggravate the systemic adverse effects of tobacco. Tobacco is generally chewed in the form of "quid," which is usually tobacco mixed with slaked lime. Tobacco products are also available in the form of gutkha and other suparis. Many people are also in the habit of rubbing a form of burnt tobacco called masheri on the teeth and gums during or after a daily dental cleaning. The local effect on the hard and soft oral tissues is undoubtedly dangerous. The place where the tobacco chewer frequently stores the "quid" is prone to develop precancerous lesions such as leukoplakia or erythroplakia. Gutkha chewing has been likened to a condition called "oral submucosal fibrosis," in which fibrous bands form in the mouth and, because of this, the oral opening is severely restricted. These precancerous conditions, if ignored and further abused with irritants, can progress to full-blown cancer. It should be noted that oral cancer has a rather poor prognosis compared to other cancers, and surgical treatment is usually quite disfiguring unless accompanied by massive surgical plastic reconstruction.

Tobacco chewers are also more likely to develop staining and discoloration of the teeth. Gums, already weakened by the local and systemic effects of tobacco, can result in pocket formation and root surface decay. Gum problems accompanied by tobacco staining also cause a distinctive breath odor and can be quite annoying to others.

The back (posterior) part of our palate contains some minor salivary glands. Cigarette smokers and other tobacco users develop the characteristic "smoker's spots" or brown spots on the roof of the mouth due to blockage of the openings of these minor glands. This condition is generally harmless, but can appear quite sinister.

The Role of Diet in Dental Health

Diet plays an important role in the prevention of tooth decay and gum disease. Factors such as the type of foods we eat, the time we eat them, and how often we eat them play an important role in the onset and progression of tooth decay and gum disease. In general, it can be said that soft, sticky, and sweet foods are bad for our teeth. One type of sugar, known as sucrose, is especially bad for our teeth. Foods with a low pH or acidic beverages, such as cold drinks, also hurt our teeth.

In general, it can be said that soft, sweet, and sticky foods are bad for teeth. In general, non-sticky and fibrous foods are good for teeth. Fibrous foods help keep the supporting tissues of the teeth healthy. They also stimulate salivary flow and promote the elimination of food from the mouth. In addition, fibrous foods are often low in extrinsic non-dairy sugars, which cause tooth decay.

Various nutritional deficiencies can hurt our teeth and gums. Deficiency of factors such as vitamin A, C, and D, calcium, and phosphorus during the stages of tooth formation can lead to defects in tooth development. Excessive intake of fluorides, or antibiotics such as tetracycline, can result in abnormal tooth shape and structure. Gum disease can be initiated or aggravated by deficiencies of substances such as folic acid, vitamin C, vitamin 812, and iron deficiency.

Dietary modification and improvement can definitely prevent dental and gum disease and improve dental and gum health. But the most important key to oral health remains regular and meticulous mechanical plaque cleaning.

CHAPTER 14:

Your Hair: Basic Hair Care Guide

H air is one of those features we take for granted. We often rush to wash our hair daily and neglect its condition... until it's too late and we find ourselves with a day of dandruff that can end with a trip to the salon. This guide will teach you some basics to keep your hair healthy, as well as some tips to combat dry ends and dandruff.

Basic Hair Care

Washing Hair with Shampoo

The shampoo is the most popular method of cleansing the hair. Simply massage some into the scalp or let it run through your fingers and then rinse. It is important to remember that washing your hair every day will strip it of all the natural oils that are designed to protect it. If you want to replace them, try olive oil or coconut oil (both of which are great for dry ends) (which can be used as a conditioning treatment).

What to look for in shampoo?

There are several factors to consider when choosing the best shampoo for your hair. The main thing is to choose one that is gentle but cleans effectively, make sure it is hypoallergenic and sulfate-free.

Avoid These Things in Your Hair

Sulfates

If your shampoo contains "sodium lauryl sulfate" or "sodium lauryl sulfate", do not use it. These products can strip away the natural oils that protect your hair, leaving it dry and brittle. If you see the words "fragrance" or "parfum" on the label, don't look. This usually means there is some type of sulfate in that shampoo.

Silicone

If your shampoo contains "dimethicone," don't use it. It coats your hair, making it feel soft and silky, but it also prevents it from absorbing its natural oils, leaving your hair dry.

Dry shampoo

The dry shampoo contains several chemicals that coat the hair, leaving it dry and feeling like a mess on your hands. It's best to wash it normally.

Sugar

Never wash your hair with sugar or any other form of granulated sugar. Sugar will clog the pores of the scalp and create more dandruff.

If your hair is oily, there are shampoos aimed at people with oily hair. If you need to combat the greasiness, keep in mind that you will need to use them daily or your problems will return.

Using Soap

It is similar to shampooing your hair. You can rinse it out or leave it on for about 15 minutes and then wash your hair as you prefer. Don't forget to lather the hair parting area for extra effect.

Using the Conditioner

Conditioner is similar to a mask; it coats the hair and retains all the natural oils, preventing them from being removed during cleansing. It is usually used after shampooing, but can also be used alone. You can either rinse out the conditioner or leave it on for about 15 minutes before shampooing, depending on your preferred method.

Coconut Oil Treatment

Coconut oil is a great way to rehydrate hair, restore shine and leave it with a smooth finish. Just take some coconut oil, rub it in your hands and then run it through your hair.

Olive Oil

Olive oil is another great way to protect your hair from the effects of shampoo. Simply take some, rub it in your hands and apply it to your hair. You can also put some in a spray bottle and spray it on after you've washed it in the shower.

Using Argan Oil

Argan oil is another great hair oil, but it also has a more distinctive argan oil smell that many people are fond of. It is important to note that if you have oily hair, argan oil will further dry out your hair making it oilier, so you will need to be careful. Apply the oil to the ends of your hair and massage for about five minutes.

Baking Soda Treatment

Baking soda is an excellent cleansing agent, so it makes sense that you can put it in your hair. You can run it through your hair or mix it with water (like shampoo) and wash your hair after 10 minutes. This treatment is good for removing product buildup, as it acts as a shampoo.

Benefits of Washing Your Hair Regularly

This may seem obvious if you have oily hair. Even if you don't have oily hair, you should wash it at least once a week to avoid product buildup. This ends up causing greasy hair and scalp breakouts.

Product buildup not only makes your hair look greasy, but it can also cause your scalp to produce extra sebum, which can be very unhealthy for your hair.

Here are some other benefits of washing your hair once a week:

1. A dry scalp contributes to the appearance of dandruff. If you have dry hair, it tends to look dull and lifeless. When you wash your hair once a week, you remove excess oil from your scalp that can contribute to dandruff. You can also find your favorite anti-dandruff treatment on the market that is specifically formulated for dry scalp. If you like shoulder-length hairstyles, you can style them in some ponytails. It is also the easiest hairstyle that makes you look fabulous in a second.

2. Washing your hair regularly will make it feel healthier. Hair generally becomes healthier when it is washed regularly, as it removes excess oil and product buildup from the hair strands, leaving the hair with a natural shine and bounce to it. Plus, when you have healthy, bouncy hair, more of it falls into place and looks very attractive.

3. Leaving hair oily or greasy is a big disadvantage for fashion-conscious girls. If you wash your hair every week, you'll be sure to remove all visible traces of product buildup and leave your hair clean and shiny. Don't get me wrong; I'm not against washing your hair once a month or so if you do. It's fine as long as you know how to manage your hair.

4. It will help you prevent dandruff and dry scalp problems. When you wash your hair, you remove excess oil and dirt from your scalp and hair strands, which can otherwise contribute to dandruff and other scalp conditions like dermatitis.

5. Gives you a healthy, natural shine. If you don't wash your hair once a week, the buildup of oil on your scalp can make it look dull and lifeless. Even if you think you wash your hair regularly, it's a good idea to wash it once a week as a precaution. Using a detangling spray can also refresh your oily locks, leaving them looking fuller and healthier.

6. Washing your hair and scalp regularly is great, as long as you use the right shampoo. Some shampoos contain harsh chemicals that can dry out the hair and leave it badly damaged.

How to Apply Conditioner

Try to apply the conditioner only to your fingertips, do not apply it to your entire hand, as this will cover your entire hand with conditioner. If you want a thicker application, put a little more on your fingers and pour the rest. When using too many hair products, make sure you don't mix them with water as this washes away the hair products and leaves hair dry and brittle. Apply conditioner from the middle of the hair downwards. Leave it on for a few minutes before rinsing it out.

How to Dry Your Hair Properly

You can use a towel or microfiber towel to dry wet hair. Don't rub your head with the towel, as this will create more oil on your scalp. Instead, run it through your hair, squeezing out the water. It is also important not to blow dry your hair too roughly with a hot blow dryer, as this can damage the cuticles.

CHAPTER 15:

Your Hair: Trimming Your Hair

I f you have healthy hair, it is important to maintain its condition by trimming the ends. Besides the fact that this will make your hair grow faster and can help with split ends, it also keeps your mane looking fresh and prevents tangles. Not only does this save you time in the morning when it comes to grooming, but it also saves you money, not to mention the time and effort of waiting for natural growth instead of taking care of it yourself.

To prepare for trimming, shower beforehand. Then use a comb to remove any tangles or knots before you start cutting. Wet hair is more difficult to manage than dry hair, so soak it in water beforehand to make it easier to handle. If you have long hair, check for places that require trimming with a rat-tail comb or other fine-toothed comb.

Use a mirror to get an exact idea of everything you need to do if it's your first time trimming your hair. Familiarize yourself with the different sections of your head, as well as how your hair falls on top. Take the scissors or clippers and start cutting just above the ear to the nape of the neck after you have a decent concept of what you are working with. Use your best judgment to make sure the situation is balanced on both sides.

Trimming According to Face Shape

Use the following guidelines to help you have the perfect trim for your face shape

- Long-faced women tend to like long cuts that end just above the shoulders. If you've never had a trimmer, this is one of the easiest ways to achieve the bald look. Start by cleaning up all the hair underneath so it's even and clean. Next, select a number two or three-blade on your trimmer and trim all but an inch of hair on each side of your head. Once you're done, take some leave-in conditioner and run it through your hair to keep it soft and smelling good.

- Round faces are much more forgiving when it comes to cutting hair because there is no specific guideline to follow. However, you should only trim the hair on the top of your head, leaving everything else alone. This is because showing too much hair below the chin will make it look bigger.

- Long hair for round faces is usually the opposite of what long hair looks like for square faces. The longer the hair, the more it will need to be trimmed to maintain its length. Choose a number three or four-blade on your trimmer, stand upright against a mirror and run it horizontally across your head from just above your ear to the nape of your neck.

- Square faces should also be trimmed evenly. The idea is to make it look smoother and less angular, so use a number two or three-blade on your trimmer. This will help remove the stray hairs that soften the edges of the face, but still, show enough length so that the hair still has volume.

- Short hair for square faces makes these faces appear more elongated, so if you have this type of look, consider keeping it long on top with a tapered back. You can also ask your hairdresser to give you a straight cut at the bottom, which could give you the appearance of sideburns.

Do-It-Yourself vs. Professional Trimming

It would be best to avoid trimming the hair yourself unless you have a lot of experience with this type of thing. You can get good advice from your stylist or from these tips we have provided. However, it would be better to have a professional do the job for you, as it will save you time, money, and stress in the long run.

Hairdressers always know where to place the clippers and how much can be removed at once. They also know how to regrow the cut quickly and naturally. You shouldn't need to do more than pop in and out of the salon once or twice a year for a trim, unless you like to change your hairstyle regularly.

CHAPTER 16:

Your Hair: Hair Care Tips

Avoid These Things to Your Hair

There are many hair care tips out there, some as old as time itself and others innovative and backed by modern science. It can be very difficult to sift through all the information available and determine what is best for your hair type.

The most important thing to keep in mind is that there is a right way and a wrong way to approach hair care. There is a right way and a wrong way to wash, dry, brush, condition, and style, and in this chapter, you will learn the right way to do these things.

Washing with Hot Water

Many people wash their hair with hot water, especially because they wash their hair during the shower and use the same temperature of the water they use for bathing, but doing this can be detrimental to the health of the scalp.

Hot water tends to dry out the scalp and this can make the hair frizzy and dry.

It is best to wash your hair with room temperature water, especially for daily washes.

Sometimes you may use products that require warmer water, but it is always better to use lukewarm water instead of hot water.

Remove excess water after washing your hair. When you finish washing your hair, use your hands to smooth your hair and remove excess water.

Rubbing with a Towel

It's best to avoid rubbing your hair with a towel to dry it. Instead, you should wrap it in a towel, and the towel will absorb excess moisture without breaking it.

Using the Hair Dryer

You probably already know this, but using a blow dryer on your hair can seriously damage it.

Blow dryers tend to damage the cuticle that houses the hair shaft. This can lead to hair breakage and stunted hair growth.

If you must blow-dry your hair, set it on the lowest setting and blow dry it until it is 70% to 90% dry, then let it dry naturally.

Direct Scalp Conditioning

Conditioning hair is usually a good idea; however, don't apply conditioner to the scalp when you do this. Instead, put conditioner in the palms of your hands, rub them together and work it through your hair from the center to the ends.

The conditioner may flatten your hair, but it will make it more lively and vibrant if you apply it at the end.

Brushing Your Wet Hair

When your hair is wet, avoid brushing it. Instead, use a stiff comb and start at the ends. Comb carefully as you work your way towards the roots so you can free all tangles without breaking or damaging the hair.

Always use natural brushes. They are much safer than plastic brushes because natural bristles help move the oils towards the ends of the hair, which helps distribute the hair's natural oils throughout the entire mane.

Nighttime Hair Care Tips

1. One of the things that put your edges at risk is friction from bed sheets and pillowcases during sleep. As you sleep, your head may rub against the pillow or bed sheets, and this friction may cause hair loss, especially around the front part of your hair. The best way to avoid this is to either use a satin pillowcase or wear a satin hair bonnet to bed at night. Satin doesn't cause friction like cotton pillowcases, so wearing a satin bonnet before using a satin pillowcase helps to prevent hair loss or breakage from friction.

2. Another thing that helps protect your hair at nighttime is tying your hair up in a loose braid. If you usually sleep on your side, you can braid one braid on each side of your hair, but if you sleep on your side, braid it in the back. This can help to prevent tangled hair, and your hair can be ready to go by morning.

3. This is especially great during the harsh winter nights. The extreme weather can dry out your hair, especially overnight. One way to keep your hair from drying out is to put a humidifier in your room at night. This is not only good for your hair, but also for your skin. Running a humidifier in your bedroom overnight helps moisturize your hair and protect your scalp while you sleep.

CHAPTER 17:

Your Hair:
Styling Tips For Beautiful Hair

A simple change of style can make your hair look better; at the very least, it can make you feel better about your hair. The styling tips below are easy to adopt, but should give you some new ways to add variety to your hairstyle. You can try any of them.

For Short Hairstyling

1. Make a side part and apply hair gel or pomade liberally. You're ready to go if you slick your hair back.

2. Ask your stylist to trim your hair with a razor blade instead of scissors to give you a tousled look.

3. To spike your short hair, rub pomade or gel on your hands and pull it straight up. It's possible that you'll be shocked at how good this appears.

4. Pixie hairstyles are very hard to grow out of. You can let the top grow long enough to pull to one side, then clip back the sides if you want to change your style without looking a mess. This will eliminate the dreadful, unattractive mullet look.

5. For a round face, you will probably look good with short hair, as long as you keep some volume on top and keep it short and tight at the bottom.

6. Get a tiny round brush and make waves while blow-drying.

7. Another good style for a round face is the long bob, also known as the lob. This is when the back is cut close to the nape of the neck, but the sides are longer. The long sides make a face appear slimmer.

For Long Hairstyling

1. A bun at the crown of the head or at the nape of the neck is a simple technique to keep long hair out of the way while also giving you a new look. Apply a small bit of leave-in conditioner to your hair near the scalp to tame those wild short hairs. Comb your hair through before tying it into a bun—no more flyaways!

2. Take a small portion of hair at each of your temples and twist it. Pin this with a bobby pin behind the ear.

3. Braid a low ponytail before twisting it into a bun at the nape of the neck and pinning it in place for a simple chignon.

4. Use bobby pins to fasten the ends of your hair under, making it look like a short bob.

5. Even if you don't have bangs, if you have long hair, you can make it look like you have bangs. Pull the layers on one side of the head across the forehead and pin them on the other side above the ear, using a bobby pin to make it look like you have side bangs.

6. Make a high ponytail with your hair and let it fall to the back of your neck and below. Catch the ponytail's hair with a long-bowed barrette and clip it to your head, right above the nape of your neck.

7. Braid your hair and weave in ribbons or strings of tiny pearls. You can spice up simple side braids, a ponytail, or a braided bun this way.

8. If you are making a ponytail, you can tighten it by pulling the hair of the ponytail to each side to cinch up the band. For one thing, pulling against the ponytail band damages the hair strands. In addition, this remedy can cause the front of your ponytail to develop unsightly lumps of uneven hair.

For Medium Hairstyling

1. Allow your hair to air dry. Take a front-row chunk of hair and twist it to the side. Weave in some ribbon and pin it behind one ear if desired. It's possible to accomplish this on one or both sides.

2. Make four braids, two on the side and two in the back. Bobby pin these in layers at the nape of the neck.

3. Make two braids, using just the hair on the top of your head. Pull the two braids back and secure them into a low ponytail, along with the rest of your hair.

4. Slip hair behind your ears and secure it with fancy combs or a barrette.

5. Longer hair, even if you want it long and don't want to cut it, still needs to be trimmed every six to eight weeks. Take off no more than a half-inch to an inch.

Tips for Manageable Curly Hair

Make your curly hair more manageable by wrapping the ends around a round brush and blow-drying them. Leave the brush until the hair on the brush cools, then pull the brush down and out. You'll have nice, manageable waves. Don't brush the hair, or the wave will be disturbed. Instead, use your fingers to push it into place.

Apply a small amount of mousse to damp curly hair and turn your head upside down. Use a diffuser on the blow dryer until the hair is 90% dry. Lift your head back up and you have a beautiful curly mane. The volume you've created will flatten out when you sleep on your hair overnight. In the morning, flip your head upside down and spritz on the dryer prep spray. It will reactivate the previous day's mousse and your hair won't look like a frizz ball.

An easy updo for curly hair is to take sections of hair about an inch thick and pin them at the nape of your neck.

Adding Style to Straight Hairs

1. People with short straight hair are in luck because they can spike their hair with product and look great.

2. If you have long straight hair, you can always pull it into a ponytail or stash it in a bun.

3. Braid portions of your hair and pull them back, fastening them behind an ear or securing them to the back of your head.

4. Straight hair is great for a fishtail braid.

5. Another interesting braiding method for straight hair is the waterfall braid. It looks intricate but is easy to make and looks amazing. Again, you'll want to search out one of several waterfall braid tutorials available on YouTube.

How to Build and Grow Your Bangs

The best brush for bangs is a small round brush with boar bristles. These bristles are close together and grab all the hairs.

Hold the blow dryer over your forehead to dry your bangs. Brush the bangs from side to side until they are completely dry. Then gently shape it with the blow dryer by running the brush underneath.

Always blow-dry your bangs right out of the shower. They dry quickly and, unless your hair is straight, you will get waves if you don't hurry.

Bangs can get a little unruly if you don't blow dry them, but there are times when you can't. If you're at the beach, you can't do it. If you're at the beach, you can't go running to dry your bangs every time they get wet. For a simple solution, part your bangs along the parting of your hair and twist them outward, pushing them to the side. Avoid touching them until they're dry; you'll see them all going in the same direction instead of being messy.

Look for the amount you put in your bangs. It's best to treat the rest of the hair first and use what's left on your hands to treat the bangs. This will prevent the bangs from looking greasy.

Avoid moisturizing your forehead except for the night before you wash your hair. Moisturizer can soak into the bangs and make them look oily.

Growing bangs is probably the most antagonistic experience you will have with your hair. You may feel like a shaggy sheepdog until it grows long enough to trim. The most elegant way to support the growth of bangs is to separate them along with the parting. If you have a side parting, sweep the bangs from that side and use hairspray to hold them in place. If you have a center parting, do a middle parting and hold it in place with hairspray or bobby pins.

1. Use a headband to keep those bangs out of your eyes until they have grown out to match the rest of your hair.

2. Pull your bangs back and fix them with a clip at the crown or slightly lower part of your head.

3. If your bangs are long enough, braid them in tiny strands and sweep them to the side, pinning them to your head.

4. Put some gel in your bangs and twist them up. Secure them with a bobby pin for a slight pompadour look.

Other Hairstyling Tips

- Did you know there was a right and wrong way to use a bobby pin? Apparently, the wavy side of the pin should be underneath, so it can grab onto your hair. The flat side remains up.

This explains a lot.

- Another tip about bobby pins is to spray them with a little hairspray before you put them in; this will give them a better grip on your hair.

- Morning hair can be a little frightening. Here is a great way to calm down that morning look and keep all those little fly-away hairs to a minimum. Get an extra toothbrush. Spray the toothbrush with hair spray and comb small sections of your hair down toward your face. This is only going to work with areas of short hair.

- If you frequently put your hair in a ponytail, don't forget to move that ponytail around from day to day to prevent the breakage of hair near the elastic band. Place the ponytail on the side of your head one day, then at the back the next. Make a high ponytail one day; the next day, make one on the side of your head or at neck's nape

- This tip can give medium-length to long hair some good volume. On the day you wash your hair, part it on one side. The next day, move the part to the other side. You will be amazed at the volume you have for two whole days.

- If your hair is full of static electricity, pull out a dryer sheet and rub it all over your hair. The static will disappear.

- Static is also controlled by rubbing a little lotion on the hands and then using the fingers to straighten the hair.

- You can wear a headband with long, medium, or short hair. Use one when you put your hair in a ponytail or bun, too. Headbands come in a variety of fabrics, including plastic; some come with a great deal of bling for a fancier look.

- Use sparkly bobby pins or ornamented hair combs to make your hair look upscale.

CHAPTER 18:

Your Body Hair

Body hair is another of the scourges of women's lives. How much easier would it be if we only had hair where we really wanted it? However, the issue needs to be addressed. All that unwanted body hair should be removed from time to time. You can choose from any of the methods listed below, depending on your preferences and budget. It should also suit your skin type, so go through them all to find the right method for you. If your goal is to remove hair permanently, you can rely on a professional esthetician to advise you which treatment is best for you.

Methods of Hair Removal

Waxing

Waxing is the way to go if you want a hair-free effect that lasts three to six weeks. Waxing may seem messy or messy, especially for coarse hair, but it's easier than you think. Smooth the strip in the direction of hair growth, hold the skin taut with one hand and pull quickly in the opposite direction with the other. If you don't remove all the hair the first time, you can use the same strip again to touch it up, which is great for the hairier sections.

Shaving

There are several myths about women and shaving. You may be particularly concerned about the following three issues:

1. Is it all right for me, a woman, to shave my face?

2. Will shaving make the hair grow back thicker?

3. Is it true that once you start shaving, you can never stop?

It's okay to shave your face, because it won't make the hair grow back thicker. This is a common misconception, but making hair thicker by shaving is a physical impossibility. The hair is dead, and there is nothing you can do to the hair above the skin that will have any effect on the living part of the hair, the follicle, below the skin. However, what does happen (and this may be why some people believe that shaving thickens hairs) is that the end of a shaved hair will be blunt and therefore the size of the full diameter of the hair (the cross-section), whereas a hair that has been allowed to grow naturally will have a tapered end that is less visible and feels softer.

It's also an old wives' tale that if you start shaving, you'll never be able to stop. Even if you don't like those blunt ends, once the hair growth cycle has passed, the blunt hairs will be replaced by tapered ones as normal.

This bluntness can make the hair feel slightly stubby, which I would say is the biggest downside for most women to shaving their face. This is unavoidable, so you'll have to weigh the slight boner against the advantages of shaving. The other disadvantage is that many women feel uncomfortable and unfeminine shaving their faces. All I can do at this point is remind you that Marilyn Monroe (along with many other historical beauties) shaved her face, and no one ever called her unfeminine.

How Often Should You Shave?

There is no right or wrong answer. Generally speaking, you should shave as often as you feel you need to, but no more than your skin can handle. For some women, this may be daily; for many, it will be once or twice a week.

First, you'll need to choose your razor: men's or women's, disposable or not. There is not much difference between men's and women's razors, except for the color. Interestingly, men's magazine articles confess that women's razors are better for men's faces because they are designed for women's contours, and women's magazine articles reveal that men's razors are better for women's bodies because they are designed for the contours of men's faces, so there really isn't going to be much difference.

As for disposable razors versus reusable razors, reusable razors have the advantage that they are usually hinged and change the angle with your contours. They will cost more, as replacement blades are more expensive than disposable razors, but you will get a better result with less skin irritation.

By the way, when a razor is disposable, it doesn't mean you have to throw it away after a single-use. It just means you should replace the entire razor after the same amount of time or number of uses as you would change the blade on a reusable razor.

If necessary, use a razor with one or two blades. Razors with six blades are frankly insane, unless you want to skin your own face.

Is shaving foam needed?

In addition to wetting your face with warm water, you will need something to lubricate. You can choose from foam, gel, cream, or oil. Foam is easy to use, as you can clearly see the areas you've shaved, but oil allows for a closer shave. The problem with oil is that it can appear to dull the blade. Actually, it doesn't dull it; it just needs to be cleaned (carefully!). You can buy a razor "sharpener" that will remove hairs, skin, and product debris, allowing you to keep using the sharp blade for longer (it doesn't actually sharpen, it just cleans, so you'll have to start with a new blade anyway). Some men use a cake of soap and a brush, but that's mostly to lift the beard hair from the skin, something women don't need to do. You can also avoid filling the basin with hot water. Unless you keep the basin obsessively clean, it won't be clean enough, and you don't need the steam to soften the hair anyway, as it won't be hard enough to require or benefit from the steam.

Change the blade whenever you feel it is dull (and cannot be sharpened again) or if you see that it is rusty. Keep your razor clean and well ventilated so that it dries properly between uses.

Shave in the direction of growth, which will help prevent ingrown hairs. If you shave in the opposite direction, you'll get a closer shave, but you're much more likely to get ingrown hairs. Some people rely on side shaving: experiment with caution if you are not satisfied with the closeness of the shave when shaving in the direction of growth. Growth can go in different directions on one part of the body (such as the neck and almost always the armpits), so you may need to shave in different directions to keep shaving in the direction of hair growth.

Is aftershaving necessary?

You don't need an aftershave, and you certainly don't want to apply cologne (both of which can irritate the skin; it never ceases to amaze me how many irritants are put in men's shaving products, such as "cooling" mint and "soothing" menthol), but you will benefit from using products on the skin after shaving to soothe the skin, discourage ingrown hairs and gently disinfect the skin. A product containing beta-hydroxy acid (BHA), also known as salicylic acid, will exfoliate pores, preventing hairs from being trapped inside. Tend Skin, a liquid with BHA, is especially good to apply after shaving. It is smelly, but the odor disappears after a few seconds.

Depilatory Creams

Depilatory cream is a home treatment that is applied to the skin and left on for a few minutes, during which time it dissolves the hair by breaking the keratin bonds, allowing the hair to be easily scraped off the surface of the skin. The active ingredient is usually calcium thioglycolate or potassium thioglycolate. It is most commonly found in cream form, but can also be found in gel, lotion, spray, or even powder form.

Depilatory creams usually have a rather unpleasant odor, which can last until the next day. The effect does not last longer than shaving. On the plus side, at least you won't be left with a sharp beard, as the hair tips don't cut as cleanly as with a razor, and some women find sitting on the edge of the bathtub with a mustache and creamy sideburns somewhat less depressing than shaving.

It's fine for areas of the body that aren't too sensitive and where you really can't tolerate stubble (like upper thighs, where stubble would rub against other areas) or if shaving just doesn't work for you, but be very careful if you use it on your face.

Polishing Pads

These are small, very rough pads, similar to sandpaper, that are rubbed in a circular motion against the skin to remove hair and exfoliate the skin. Because they are abrasive to the skin, they can only be used once a week, at which time the hair will become visible again. They work best on fine hair, as if the hair is coarser, you may have to scrub so hard to remove the hair that the skin is raw, but where the hair is finer (probably the face), the skin is delicate and may not tolerate buffing.

The main advantages of epilating with a buffer are that there is no stubble (because, unlike shaving, epilating with a buffer does not leave a clean cross-section of hair) and that it can be less emotionally uncomfortable than shaving the face. Ingrown hairs are also avoided since you exfoliate while epilating.

The disadvantages are the duration, that it does not work for everyone or on all areas of hair, that the skin may be sore from the procedure, and that the results are no longer lasting than shaving, but cannot be repeated as often.

Obviously, people with sensitive skin should proceed with caution, if at all. And just in case you were thinking about it: please don't try your own cheap version using real sandpaper, as regular sandpaper has much sharper edges on the sand particles and can scratch your skin.

Bleaching

This is not, strictly speaking, hair removal, of course, but an alternative method of disguising hair.

Frankly, I think it's of limited use, especially on the face: a blond mustache is still a mustache and is not significantly less visible than a dark one. In fact, if you have dark or tanned skin, blond hair will stand out just as much as dark hair on light skin, since the contrast is the same. In addition, it is a big hassle for a procedure that does not remove any hair, and can still irritate the skin. Dark skin, in particular, may be temporarily lightened by the treatment for a few days. The results will not last long, as any regrowth will be the original color of the hair.

On the plus side, there is no stimulation of growth, there should be no pain, no stubble, and no ingrown hairs. It's a decent option for some very specific circumstances: for example, arm hair is generally considered acceptable in a way that most female body hair is not (and hairless arms can look strange since we're not as used to seeing them as hairless legs), but you may feel that your arm hair is too dark, in which case bleaching would leave the hair present but make it more subtle.

Alternative Removal Methods

- Alkaline wash

- Medications

- Birth control pills

- Homemade Anti-androgen treatments

CHAPTER 19:

Your Fragrance: Overview

Almost everyone likes to smell good. In fact, we not only want to smell good on the inside, but also on the outside. We want our clothes to smell nice and leave a pleasant aroma, as well as enjoy the scent of perfume and cologne.

There is no doubt that fragrance can turn a bad day into a day we will remember for all the right reasons. Whether it's the aroma of freshly baked goods wafting down the street or the smell of tropical fruits and flowers as we stroll through an exotic garden, all smells make us happy, and some even make us feel good.

Fragrances are more than just scents; they also say something about us as individuals. Our sense of smell plays an important role in our sense of self and how we perceive ourselves. Scent has the added benefit of allowing us to connect with others through scent transfer. This is especially true in the case of lovers or friends; whether they realize it or not, everyone can detect their partner's distinctive scent.

Smells, like taste and sight, can be interpreted and perceived through a variety of methods.

Adding Scent to Your Skin

Many people may think that adding a scent to the skin is simply impossible. In fact, there are several ways to add it. While many of us are familiar with diffusing essential oils, few know that they can also be added to the skin. How you do this depends on the oil or oils you choose to use, but diffusing them before or after is always a good idea.

Here are some general pointers to...

1. Adding essential oils to the skin is best done with a carrier oil

2. You have multiple options for how you can add the scent

3. Some essential oils are better for certain uses than others

4. You can create custom blends

5. These blends will change over time

6. Be careful with the choice of your oils

7. Don't use essential oils with babies or children, especially before bedtime

8. Always seek professional guidance before using essential oils on the skin.

Adding Scent to Your Clothing

One of the best ways to get an idea of what you're wearing is with a trusted nose. But what if you can't get close enough to your clothes or they don't smell? Body odor is not the only reason we can have bad smells. The smell of our clothes and hair also influences our odor.

In addition to washing well and applying fabric conditioners, you can try these five simple tips to perfume your clothes.

1. Perfume spray - The easiest way to quickly spruce up a garment is with a perfume spray if you have one handy. All you have to do is spray a little on the inside of your clothes, and they're ready to go. If you don't have a perfume spray, then a little hairspray or any scented body spray will also work well.

2. Scrubs - If you have body scrubs lying around, it's very simple. Just massage the scrub particles onto your clothes to give them a subtle scent. If you have a whole jar of scrubs, rub them all over your clothes.

3. Lotion - The best way to add your own scent to clothing is with a little lotion. Cheap body lotions come in a variety of scents, so if you don't have any around the house, use one that smells good and that you think you'll enjoy using.

4. Perfume Oils - This is a great option for anyone who has a perfume room in their home. Perfume oils are relatively inexpensive and easy to make at home. All you have to do is pour a small amount of perfume into a small glass bottle with a dropper.

5. Vinegar - If you have vinegar at home, this is probably the cheapest option. Just soak your clothes in vinegar, and they will give off a scent after drying.

Adding Scent to Your Hair

Here are the ways to add scent to your hair without the use of strong perfumes.

1. Put your shampoo into a spray bottle, then add a few drops of essential oils. Before use, give it a good shake to disperse the oils evenly throughout the liquid. It will be easier for your hair to absorb the scents if you do this.

2. Apply a few drops of essential oil directly into the palm of your hand and rub it all over your hair. Then apply the oil to a small section on each side of the head. Depending on how much oil you add, your hair may be a bit greasy the next day.

3. Take a handful of shampoo and then add in a few drops of the essential oils that you want to smell like. Massage onto your hair and scalp. Hang for a few minutes before rinsing.

4. Boil some water, infuse the essential oils in it, and then apply to your dry hair. Before rinsing, leave the shampoo on for at least 5 minutes.

5. To make a DIY conditioner, combine essential oils with a conditioner. Before rinsing, apply the conditioner to your hair and keep it on for a few minutes.

6. Create a sweet-smelling dry shampoo. Put a handful of dry shampoo into a mason jar. Add a few drops of essential oil and pour in some water. Shake the bottle well before each use for oils to evenly distribute through the product.

CHAPTER 20:

Your Fragrance: About Perfumes

Perfume is essential for our health and our social life. Perfumes are manufactured by many famous brands found in stores, but they are also handmade by the people of the neighborhood.

Perfume is not only a luxury thing, because it is useful for our health and it is pleasant to wear in social life. Perfume can be bought in department stores, or it can be made in many homes or neighborhoods that have this ability to create perfumes.

Popular Perfume Scents

Many people don't know, but there are different types of perfume. There are fruity, floral, and aquatic perfumes that can be long-lasting or concentrated. You can find your favorite type of perfume by knowing the difference between these three categories and which one you like best.

Fruity

The first category is fruity. If you like this type of perfume, it will have a sweet smell reminiscent of fruits or berries. These perfumes can be found in major department stores and high-end boutiques.

Floral

The next type is the floral perfume. This perfume will undoubtedly smell like flowers or herbs. You can find this type in department stores, but this type of perfume is usually quite expensive due to the complexity of its ingredients.

Aquatic

This type of perfume smells like clean water. It is the most popular perfume among women, and it always smells great because it is long-lasting and subtle at the same time.

Perfume on Different Occasions

Fragrances are not just for everyday use; they are also great for special occasions. Now that you know that there are different perfumes for different occasions, it's time to find out what they are. There are perfumes for all kinds of events. It is also essential to keep in mind the points mentioned above on how to choose the right fragrance. This will help you choose the perfect perfume for every occasion.

Here are the different perfumes for occasions:

- **Sports Perfume**

- **Perfume for Formal Use**

- **Perfume for Dating**

- **Perfume for Special Occasion**

Choosing the Right Perfume for You

There is a lot of controversy about what perfume to wear. Is it too strong? Too light? What does someone next to you think of the scent you wear? Should you wear something for yourself or for your partner?

As we age, our sense of smell diminishes, making it hard to tell if people like our perfume. Don't be offended if there are a bunch of guys telling you they like your perfume when in reality, they don't (but I'm not trying to make any personal attacks here). You can't smell yourself, and others can't smell you. This makes it hard to tell if your perfume is too strong or not strong enough.

The first thing you should do is test the perfume by spraying it on a handkerchief or tissue, not on your bare skin. You should make sure you don't have any allergies to the perfume ingredients before applying them directly to your skin. If you are not allergic, choose a spot on your forearm and spray the perfume there. Wait ten minutes and smell the spot without washing it using only your nose (not your hands). Make sure that during this time you are NOT wearing any cologne, deodorant, or scented lotion. You want to know what you will smell like if someone hugs you or snuggles against you. If it's too firm, choose a lighter scent.

The other important thing to consider when choosing a perfume is the situation (or situations) you're going to wear it in. If you're going out on the town, to clubs and bars, look for something light and fruity with notes of rose or lily (like Chanel No. 5). This will help mask any unpleasant odors (such as alcohol or tobacco smoke) that may be on your skin. A perfume with strong citrus notes (such as orange blossoms) will give you an aura of energy and make you look younger. If you're looking for a more serious relationship, something with notes of amber or musk can make you look more mature while still smelling sweet.

Conversely, if you're facing an interview, presentation, school project, or other stressful situation, choose something more seductive. Choose a perfume that is not too sweet. The last thing you want is to smell like dessert. Choose something with a hint of spice (like cinnamon, clove, or tonka bean). Choose something with oriental notes if you want to make a more professional impression (like sandalwood).

The third criterion to keep in mind is the age of the person or people who will be smelling your perfume. If you are a young woman looking to attract older men, choose something with notes of aldehydes and moss. The sweetness of these notes will make you smell younger and less mature. This makes it seem less likely that you've been around the block a few times. This also goes for men looking to attract younger women, but in this case, they want to smell more manly and sensual than sweet and cozy. Choose a base note of leather, musk, or tobacco. Sweet notes will seem too childish.

Make sure that if you are going to buy a fragrance for someone else, you know their preferences. If you want to smell older, choose something with sandalwood notes. If you want to attract younger men and women, choose a sweet, fruity scent. If they're looking for a serious relationship (which may or may not go anywhere), opt for something that makes them think of your favorite place in the world while still smelling like fun and passion.

Once you've made your selection and figured out what works best for your environment, be sure to wear it sparingly (never more than three sprays).

How Stronger and Longer the Scent Should Be?

How strong should the perfume be? That depends on who you are targeting. A good rule of thumb is to use the three "s" rule: the more people around, the better, and the more skin you want to cover, the stronger the perfume should be. This is not to say that you should overdo it, because the human sense of smell can be trained. If you are always in public, consider an upward scent curve most of the time. After a while, people will get used to it and stop paying attention.

People perceive perfume differently, and everyone has their own way of getting used to perfume. Waiting until your company leaves and no longer notices your perfume can also help you understand if the perfume is too strong for you.

If you're looking for a scent that lasts all day, opt for a soft, subtle fragrance. If you want to use a scent that lasts as long as possible, some specific types of fragrances will help you achieve this. Be sure to check the ingredients well, as anything containing alcohol will be stronger than those containing fresh essences and essential oils.

If you like the smell of a perfume, but it doesn't last long, you can also try mixing two different fragrances to get an even more unique scent. If you wear the same perfume every day, try switching it up to keep things fresh and interesting. If you wear perfume in public, people will eventually get used to it and stop recognizing the scent.

If you really like perfume, but it doesn't last long on your body, you can try spraying it on your clothes instead of your skin. The scent will last longer there than on the skin, so if you find that the scent is too strong for you, don't worry. Just wear something close to where you are going to be all day.

The duration varies depending on the weather and climate you live in. When it's hot, all perfumes last longer, while when it's cold, they last less.

CHAPTER 21:

Your Eye: Eyebrows And Eyelashes

Your Eyebrow

Eyebrows frame the eyes and can make or break a look.

There are different eyebrow shapes that everyone should desire. The ideal eyebrow shape is a combination of the following: straight and long, thick and arched, and symmetrical. Some say the triangular shape is more flattering than others, as it can frame the eyes well and create a more balanced look. And then there are the dramatic eyebrow shapes, which are best suited for movie stars or beauty queens who want to make an impact with their facial features.

Different Shapes of Eyebrow

Here are the different shapes of eyebrow shapes that can make us look more stunning and beautiful:

Angled Brows

Angled eyebrows are the most common. It is ideal for those who have an oval face shape, as it can give a well-defined face. Angled eyebrows are great for those who want to highlight the eyes for a bright and alert look.

Arched Eyebrows

Arched eyebrows are best suited for round or square faces. It is one of the most popular eyebrow shapes because it balances the facial features very well. An arched eyebrow can make even the smallest eyes appear brighter.

Rounded Eyebrows

A slightly rounded shape is best suited for those with oblong faces. It is easy to maintain and looks very natural. This type of brow shape can make you look older, but not daintily so.

Thick, Arched Eyebrows

Thick and arched eyebrows are good for those who want to highlight their eyes and draw more attention to them. It is best suited for people with long and oval faces. It is elegant and beautiful, and can make an ordinary look more dramatic.

Straight Eyebrows

Straight eyebrows are ideal for those who want to highlight their eyes, as there is nowhere else for the light to reflect. Straight eyebrows are also ideal for people who have small eyes and short, round faces. It can add a dramatic effect to the overall look of the face. It makes you look younger and more sophisticated. Asian girls are fans of straight eyebrows, and it is one of their secrets to look younger and rejuvenated than their age.

Symmetrical Eyebrows

Symmetrical eyebrows are naturally attractive to anyone, and it's also the easiest thing to maintain. The ideal symmetrical eyebrow shape is a straight line that starts from the middle of the forehead and ends at the center of the eye. It can give a more youthful look, but not unnaturally so.

Steps on How to Shape Your Brows

For many women, brow shaping and tweezing is a surprisingly time-consuming and tedious process. Here's how it's done:

If this is the first time you want to have your eyebrows shaped, we recommend that you use the wax only on the lower arch of the eyebrow. This way you can get an idea of the shape you like and you will avoid unsightly marks if you pluck them too soon.

We recommend that you go to a hairdresser for this or, if you feel confident enough, try it yourself with tweezers.

Be sure to set aside a good hour to get the job done.

- **Step 1:** Remove any stray brow hairs with your tweezers or razor.

- **Step 2:** Carefully comb back the brows to get them in their natural position, and use your tweezers to pluck out any stray hairs that are out of place.

- **Step 3:** Brush your eyebrows with a brow brush to get them off the hairspray or gel that you used to tame them.

- **Step 4:** Apply brow powder over the entire arch of the brows to help keep them in place.

You should look for clean lines to define your natural arch and shape it at a 60° angle that takes into account the natural curve where your nose meets your face.

Your Eyelashes

Eyelashes are a key factor in human beauty because they create a desired contrast to the surrounding skin and eyes.

They also serve to protect the eye from external aggressions; for example, if someone has long eyelashes, they are more likely to protect their eyes from dirt and/or pollution.

In addition, it has long been known that the most beautiful people are those with long eyelashes that reach beyond the eyebrows.

How to Grow Your Eyelashes?

Powdering

Are you tired of doing things the old-fashioned way when it comes to your eyelashes? Did you know that powdering your eyebrows can help them grow faster and fuller? Here's how to do it quickly and easily. Just follow these simple steps and you'll see how your long-neglected lashes start to turn around and greet you with sensual charm.

Powder your lashes every day after cleansing to help achieve fuller, faster growth. Plus, it will keep your mascara from clumping or fading too quickly.

You will need: A large bottle of moisturizing mascara, a small mesh strainer, a mixing bowl, and a spoon.

In a small bowl, mix one-part mascara and three parts cream with a spoon. Apply a thin layer of the mixture to your lashes and coat them with a thin layer of mascara. It's best to use a waterproof or colored mascara if you can find one that lasts longer than four hours. Use your fingers to pull the lashes from both sides and make sure they don't get tangled.

Castor Oil

Castor oil is the best natural emollient for eyelashes. It increases eyelash growth and thickness by 20 percent, says cosmetic chemist Jutta Renger. "You have to use castor oil because it absorbs quickly into the eyelashes."

As an important factor, it can strengthen both the roots and the capillaries of your hair. If you opt to use this ingredient, make sure you use a pure product that contains little or no solvents or harsh chemicals, according to Renger.

The Idea of Fake Eyelashes

These days, false lashes are everywhere, and it's hard to have a makeup look without them. From runway models to your favorite celebrity on the red carpet, going for a ripped look is practically a rite of passage. But before you get carried away with the glamour of these Hollywood-approved accessories, answer this question first: do you have sensitive eyes?

In some cases—especially when you have particularly sensitive eyes—it may not be safe to wear false lashes. The adhesive used to hold them in place can sometimes cause uncomfortable irritation and dryness. So before you try a new pair, test them on the back of your hand first. If you're confident that they come in contact with your skin, you should be prepared.

When you finally get your hands on a pair of false eyelashes, there are a few things to keep in mind before you use them.

Here are some tips for those who want to know how to wear it effectively:

1. Always clean the glue off the lash strip with a tissue. The last thing you want is a smudge on your eye, so be sure to clean it right away.

2. Wait for 3-4 minutes to let it dry before wearing it. When you apply a lash, be sure to put it on slowly and gently so that you won't accidentally rip off your lashes while moving around.

3. Choose the right size of false eyelashes to suit your face. It should be the right size to completely cover your natural lash line without being too big or bulky.

4. Apply mascara before putting on fake lashes to ensure a better application and a more attractive look. With a few coats of mascara, your lash line will blend more naturally with the fakes, and you won't have to worry about it looking too sparse away from the center of your eyelid.

5. Always apply the adhesive only on the lash strip and not on your natural lashes. This will avoid any messy mistakes and ensure a better look for you once you're done.

6. If using an eyelash curler, curl your natural lashes first before applying fake lashes to ensure a better look for your eyes. A lash curler can also be used to give your artificial eyelashes more volume, making them appear bigger and thicker when worn.

7. If your fake lashes are longer than your natural lash line and you want to trim them, be sure to trim them so that the lashes fall above the crease of the eye. This will help them blend in more naturally with your natural lashes and create a more natural look.

8. When removing fake eyelashes, be sure to use a mild oil such as jojoba or castor oil to remove the adhesive. Avoid using makeup remover, which is too harsh for your natural eyelashes.

9. If you want as many lashes as your heart's content, then it's best to invest in a lash adhesive that allows you to reuse your fake lashes for as long as possible. This way, you can use each pair multiple times without having to be apprehensive about them running out soon.

10. Always be sure to thoroughly clean your fake eyelashes before replacing them. This will ensure that you won't have any adhesive that gets onto your lashes when you remove them. It's highly recommended that you never reuse fake lashes because of the risk of exposing yourself to hepatitis A through sharing used adhesive.

With these tips, you'll be on your way to beautiful, thick lashes like the stars. Wear them with pride and confidence - who says having perfect eyes is out of reach?

Always remember that while false lashes can give the illusion of length and volume to your eyes, they are not a substitute for proper makeup application techniques. It is best to apply mascara over false lashes to highlight their presence on your eyes and give them a more natural look.

CHAPTER 22:

Your Eye: Eye Makeups

Eyeliners

The eyeliner is an integral part of any makeup application. Eyeliner brings the eyes into focus with the rest of the facial features without overpowering them.

Different Types of Eyeliner

- Pencil eyeliners are the most common. The constant sharpening can bother you, but they're great for getting precise color right where you want them on the lash lines. Easy to handle, soft pencils can be subtle or bold.

- Liquid or gel eyeliners are difficult to use when they come in long handles, with the brush tip instead of the pen-like form. It dries very quickly, so be snappy in blending.

- Cream eyeliners are easy to apply and give intense color, but they come with a brush applicator that you have to wash after every application to prevent waxing on the bristles.

Color Choices

It complements your hair color and your eyes. Blacks, grays, browns, and navy blues are foolproof for everyone and very easy to match with eye shadow. In general, bronze and gold tones go well with blue eyes. Brown eyes go with purples and creams. Browns and intense green colors, such as sage and emerald, highlight green eyes.

How to Apply

1. If possible, lean your elbow on a flat surface to give your hand steady support.

2. Pencils can be used instantly for brushes, prime with liquid, gel, or cream eyeliner. You might have to go for a second dip later.

3. Look down. Draw a line as close as possible to your lash line. Start from the inner corner of your eye and stroke toward the center of your lid. Begin again from the outer corner (with a fresh dip from the cream/liquid/gel, if you're using that formula) and meet the existing eyeliner in the middle.

4. Use a sponge tip to evenly blend the eyeliner into your lash line.

5. Line your lower lid next. Start from the outer corner this time. Your line should go thinner as it goes to the inner corner of your eye.

Eye Shadow

Eye shadow, along with eyeliner, can transform your entire face. It makes eyes look bigger and enhances their color, giving you a bright and seductive look.

Different Types of Eye Shadow

- **Powder Eye Shadow:** The compact of pressed powder is divided into two, three, or four colors. Powder eye shadow is very easy to apply and can be blended wet or dry with a sponge tip or brush.

- **Cream Eye Shadow:** This comes in small or large compacts, like watercolor palettes we used as kids. Cream formulation eye shadow lasts longer than powder eye shadow. It's also easy to apply with a brush or finger. Unless it's oil-control or mattifying, cream eye shadow is not recommended for women with oily skin.

- **Liquid Eye Shadow:** Liquid eye shadow comes in tubes or tubs, in one color or two. It is often smudged and waterproof. The pigments cleave to the skin, which makes this ideal to wear for outdoor activities and water activities where you'll sweat or get wet. It is also very easy to apply with a sponge or finger.

Color Choices

Our eyelids already have a natural pigmentation. Look in the mirror: they can have a hint of brown, gray, pink, or purple. Browns and taupe flatter all eye colors and complexions because they are the most natural shades. The same goes for lavender; just keep in mind to apply this color very sparingly to avoid a bruised look.

For the other eye shadow colors, keep in mind your hair color and go close to it. Contrasting it too drastically will make you look pale or raccoon. For example, if you have light hair, choose light, pastel colors for your eyeshadow. If you have dark hair, you can opt for intense shades.

Aside from grays and taupe shades, which are always sure bets for everyone, these are the colors you want for that color-pop effect:

1. **For blue or gray eyes** – Pinks, deep reds, and orange shades

2. **For green or hazel eyes** – Purples and browns with sunny yellow or gold undertones

3. **For brown eyes** – So many colors to choose from! Try them all out. Consider your hair color for maximum effect. Amber and lavender shades are for brown-eyed gals with light hair. Darker, deeper colors of gray and purplish hues are for brown eyes paired with dark hair.

Applicator Choices

Brushes come in different sizes and shapes, depending on their use. Eyelid brushes are rounded, while those for the corners and creases of the eyes are narrow and angled for precision. Tips are also flat, rounded, or angled. Natural bristles always last longer and are better for blending than synthetic bristles.

1. **Flat, stiff brush** – used mainly to layer color on the eyelids. Its tip can also be used as a liner for the lower lids.

2. **Pencil brush** – the pointed tip is great for intensifying color on the corners of the eyes or applying

3. **Dome brush** – the stiff and soft varieties offer precision contouring, blending, and softening of colors.

Sponge tips come with pressed compact powder eyeshadow, and apply colors vibrantly in one or two coats, but you'll need the help of a brush to avoid sharp color lines.

Fingertips are best for cream eyeshadow. The warmth of our touch softens the cream and helps to blend and smooth it easily over our eyelids.

How to Apply

When you're going to apply eyeshadow, you should be wearing foundation and primer. And if you're wearing either of these two, you should have already cleansed, toned, and moisturized, right?

1. Use an eye primer and coat your eyelids evenly. Let it set.

2. Choose two to three shades of color –light, medium, and dark. The lighter shade becomes a highlighter and provides a contrast for the darker shades to stand out. If you want dark eyes, you start with light shades, and so on.

3. For the classic smoky look: pack dark color on top of your eyelid and go medium to light as you work up to the brow bone, softening the dark shade. The darkest color should never reach past the crease of your eye.

4. To open up eyes and make them appear larger, apply your light shade to the inner corner (around the tear ducts).

5. If you use a quad palette, the fourth shade is shimmery rather than matte, and this is what it's meant for, as an "eye-opener" for the inner corner or just under your eyebrows.

6. In contrast, the outer corner of the eye should be dark.

7. For another look, use your light shade in the inner corner, the medium shade at the center of your eye, and the dark shade at the outer corner of your eye.

8. Blend well. This is the golden rule of eye shadow application. There shouldn't be defined lines of color.

Mascara

Mascara is like a magic wand: it takes your look from drab to fabulous, even if you don't apply any other makeup! Many women don't leave home without mascara. Wearing mascara is like opening wide the windows and letting those beautiful curtains flutter.

Different Types of Mascara

1. **Volumizing** – This formulation is the best for a heightened dramatic look and dark eyes, even without eyeliner or eyeshadow. Volumizing mascara thickens lashes and gives an illusion of fullness through waxes and silicone polymers that coat each strand and build your lashes up.

2. **Lengthening** – This formulation is for women with short and sparse lashes. Lengthening mascara gives you more by extending your lashes through fibers that attach at the end of the strands.

3. **Curling** – This formulation adds curls to your lashes, of course. It opens, defines, and highlights your eyes while thickening your lashes for a very flattering look.

4. **Waterproof** – This is perhaps the best-selling formulation because you don't have to worry about crying, swimming, or simply leaking up from an eye irritation while out for the day. Eyes are wet, after all, and waterproof mascara stays on and does its magic despite tears or sweat.

Color Choices

1. There are not a lot of color options for mascara unless you want to look like a visitor from outer space.

2. Black mascara is the most natural and flattering look. It's perfect for everyone, from blondes to brunettes. Black displays length and volume best, not to mention it adds color-popping qualities for your eyes.

3. Brown mascara also looks nice for fair-haired and red-haired women. For brunettes, black brings out the eyes.

4. Bright mascara colors like purples, greens, and blues should be left for runway models and teenagers to test out.

Brush Choices

1. **The right mascara is applied to its fullest potential using the right brush. If you have long lashes** – lucky you – you need a thicker brush. For shorter lashes, go for a short-bristled brush.

2. **Straight brush** – is always versatile and in-demand because it's easy to use and gives you solid access to your eye corners.

3. **Curved brush** – is for making natural-looking curls.

4. **Comb** – helps in de-clumping and lash separation. Combs come straight or curled.

5. **Spherical brush** – lets you decide how much formula you want on your lashes so you can increase the boldness bit by bit.

How to Apply

1. Always use a curler first. This little tool does wonders to your eyes. Just be careful to clamp on eyelashes, not your eyelid.

2. Twist the wand back and forth within the tube instead of pushing it in and out to get an adequate amount of mascara on the brush. Pumping the brush will merely introduce air bubbles into the solution, causing it to dry out and clump.

3. As with eyeliner, lean your elbow on a surface if you can.

4. Never apply mascara before powdering around your eyes, and never apply mascara over the top of your eyelashes. This will weigh your eyelashes down, and they'll close over your eyes! Mascara is applied from underneath the upper eyelash.

5. Place the brush/comb of your mascara wand to the roots of your eyelashes and wiggle the bristles back and forth a little to get the product on the base of the hair strands. Mascara at the roots, rather than the tips, is what gives the illusion of length.

6. Work from the base to the tips, rolling the wand as you go. This separates the lashes and avoids clumping.

7. To further distribute and separate your lashes, run a comb from the roots to the tips.

8. As you wait for this first coat to dry on your upper eyelashes, apply mascara on your lower ones. Use a very light hand here because hair is sparse, and you don't want to smudge the product onto your skin after working hard with a concealer to make that part of your face light!

9. After a minute or two, the eyelashes are ready for a second coat. Some mascara products enable you to pile it on until you achieve your desired volume and drama. Cheaper mascara just clumps if you apply too much, so watch for clumping as you apply each coat.

CHAPTER 23:

Your Make-Up: An Overview

Beauty is fashion; fashion is art. Makeup can be used to enhance natural features or to create a whole new face for any occasion. In addition, beauty tips are not only vital for maintaining healthy skin, but are also essential for achieving an airbrushed effect that leaves skin looking flawless. This is because makeup, in all its forms, can be used to cover imperfections and improve the overall appearance of the skin.

Different Types of Makeup

You're going to need makeup for an upcoming night out and you're not quite sure which type of makeup will best suit your needs. Even if you know the purpose of each type of makeup, it can be difficult to determine which one is right for you.

Here are the most popular types on the market today, available in both drugstores and department stores.

Concealer

Concealers come in a wide range of forms, from high-intensity foundation to light foundation. They are intended to cover minor imperfections and are useful for everyday or special occasions. For best results, apply with a sponge or brush around the affected area. Do not use on top of foundation.

Foundation

Foundation offers great coverage, but is usually distinguished from concealer by its thickness and creamy texture. It is available in liquid, powder, stick, and cream forms. Coverage starts at light, depending on the type.

Powder

Pressed powder is translucent or white in color. Its texture is similar to cream makeup, and it is ideal for covering skin imperfections, such as pimples and blemishes. Consider applying concealer afterward if you want to minimize blemishes.

Lipstick

Rub lips with your lipstick or lip gloss of choice to give them a hint of color before applying foundation or powder for the most natural-looking result. Apply an opaque lip color two to three shades lighter than your natural lip color.

Lip Liner

A lip liner helps create perfect lips by leaving a small amount of color around the outside of your lips. To do this, apply it with a liquid liner or liquid liner brush. Be sure to use a soft, fluffy brush so you can deposit enough product on the areas you want to cover without applying too much at once. Do not apply directly to the lips.

Blush

The blusher comes in cream, powder, and gel form and works much like foundation in that it provides great coverage for imperfections, such as skin blemishes. It comes in a variety of colors and is one of the best types of makeup to use if you're looking for a more natural look.

Bronzer

Bronzer gives your face an extra glow and can be used to add color to areas of the face, such as the cheeks or forehead. It is less covering than blusher, but can be used to create a more natural look with less product.

Highlighter

Illuminator is a powder that makes skin appear brighter and can add a luminous look if used in the right places. It is usually applied with a brush or fingers to areas such as the cheekbones and inner corners of the eyes, but can also be applied over the foundation to give the face a natural glow.

CHAPTER 24:

Your Make-Up:
Sample Make-Up Routine

A makeup routine is a set of steps that a woman follows to achieve the desired effects for her face and body. These routines vary in length and may include different types of makeup, such as lipstick, foundation, blusher, eye shadow, etc.

You can follow the following steps for your makeup. Remember that you can also plan your own makeup routine, depending on your personal preferences and skin type.

Moisturizer

1. Prep your skin with a moisturizer

2. Start by spreading the moisturizer across your forehead; begin from the center of your face, then move outwards and up.

3. Repeat the procedure starting at your nose, spreading the moisturizer across your cheeks.

4. Gently rub the moisturizer in using circles

5. Dry before applying the primer

Primer

1. Apply a small amount of primer by squeezing it onto your fingertips or onto a makeup brush or sponge

2. Work the primer from the center of your face towards your forehead, cheeks, and chin.

3. Start with a small amount of primer in the center of your face. Then slowly work it out towards your cheeks, forehead, and chin.

Liquid Foundation

1. Using either your finger or a makeup brush/sponge, you may now apply the liquid foundation

2. Start from the center of your face and blend the liquid foundation outwards.

3. As you sweep your foundation across the skin, be sure to buff it in.

4. Stipple a damp sponge over its foundation to assist it is seeping into the lines and creases, resulting in a smoother, more similar texture.

Concealer

1. Apply the light concealer beneath the eyes with a damp sponge or makeup brush.

2. Apply the concealer to the areas where blemishes appear. (optional)

3. Highlight the face using a liquid or cream concealer by placing small dots horizontally over the center of your forehead down to the center of your nose

4. Next, place small dots under your eyes in a curving arch at the top of your chin, just under your bottom lip

5. Gently blend to the surrounding skin. Make sure to cover with a foundation or setting powder.

Foundation Powder

1. Using a large powder brush, dust a light coat of foundation powder all over your face.

2. Press the bristles into the powder, then sweep across the skin in long, arching strokes.

3. You may apply a bit more powder on the red and oily areas of your face as an option. Be sure to press the powder firmly onto the skin for the powder to penetrate the pores and lines to create a smooth skin texture.

Bronzer

1. Using a bronzer brush, apply a bronzer across your face. Familiarity in choosing the right shade is essential in this matter

2. Apply your bronzer in the shape of a number "3" on both sides of the face.

3. Pull the bronzer across your cheekbones, then across your jawline, all the way down to your chin, starting at your forehead.

Blush

1. Blush can be applied as an option to increase the vibrancy of your complexion.

2. Using a dense brush with many bristles, apply your blush, making sure you get the most out of every blush sweep. It's your preference on what of blush to choose

Highlighter

1. Complement your makeup with the right highlighter. Map out the areas you wish to highlight. You can choose between a liquid, cream, or powdered highlighter.

2. Apply a liquid highlighter in these areas of your face

- Down the bridge of your nose

- Across the tops of your cheekbones

- Inner corners of your eyelids

- The indent above your upper lip

- The center of your forehead and chin

- On your brow bone

3. Blend now your highlighter using your fingertips or a sponge

Eye Shadow

1. Dip your eyeshadow brush into the light shade, then tap the brush to get rid of any excess product.

2. Apply the lighter shadow across the entire lid, starting at the lash line and ending just above the crease of your eyelid.

3. Now dip your brush into the darker hue and tap off any excess. Apply the color to the outer corner of your eye, just above your lash line. Sweep the darker color just behind the brow bone, over the crease of your eyelids.

4. Stop application around the center of your eyelid, as you don't want to darken the inner corners.

5. Blend the two shades together with a clean shadow brush. Reapply the darker shadow if you want an even more vivid appearance.

Eyeliner

1. Apply now the liquid eyeliner working thin at the inner corner of your eye the thicker towards the outer corner. Begin lining your eyes in the center, keeping the liner tip or brush as close to the lash line as possible.

2. Create little dashes down the lash line with small strokes of your liner, then join them to fill in the spaces. Don't worry if your hand slips!

3. Eyeliners in other forms (gel and pencil) can also be applied as an alternative.

Mascara

1. Before applying mascara, make sure to curl your eyelashes:

- Close the curler slowly at the base of your upper lashes, taking care not to grab any of the delicate skin around your eyelid.

- Hold it for a few seconds before gently releasing it.

- Grab your mascara tube once you've curled your eyelashes. Gently swirl the wand to coat all of the bristles in mascara.

- Lightly wriggle the mascara brush through the roots of your lashes. This will give your lashes more volume, which you may then pull through to the ends.

- If your lashes have clumped together, take a clean wand and brush them through.

- For added volume, apply a second coat.

2. Make now a few swipes of mascara to make your eyes look brighter

Lip Gloss

1. Before you apply gloss, make sure your lips are clean. If your lips are dry and cracked, use a light lip scrub to exfoliate any dead skin.

2. To soften the lips, even more, apply a lip conditioner or moisturizer. Blot any extra lip balm after it has been absorbed.

3. Apply your lip gloss now, starting in the middle of your lips and dragging the applicator along the length of your pout. Avoid drawing any gloss above your natural lip line, and lightly press your lips together to ensure that your lip gloss reaches all of your lips' nooks and crevices.

Setting

1. Making a final touch by applying setting spray or setting powder can be the final touch for your makeup routine. Setting pray is similarly applied to you as hairspray. Spray while holding the bottle at least 8 inches away from your face.

Your makeup is now complete.

It's easy to create a range of beauty looks with these makeup application tips, whether you're headed to the office or out for a night on the town.

CHAPTER 25:

Your Make-Up: Fabulous Make-Up Tips

Make-Up Tips Based on Face Shapes

Makeup that looks good on an oval face may not suit you if you have a square face. When choosing and applying makeup we take into account skin type, skin tone, and hair color. We must not forget the shape of our faces!

For Square Face

The square face usually has an angular jawline and a wide forehead to match. It can be softened with a haircut with bangs or angular layers on one side of the face.

- Keep your brows rounded and curving rather than straight.

- Apply a highlighter on the center of your forehead, chin, and cheekbones. These shimmery spots will draw attention to the center of your face rather than the angular sides and corners.

- Make use of shading – use a dark foundation or a bronzer to minimize the impact of strong jaws.

- The shading trick also goes for your blush. Apply a darker shade on the hollow of your cheeks, brushing upward, followed by a lighter shade over your cheekbones. Blend well! Make sure any distinct lines made by two different colors are brushed so that the distinction is subtle.

- To create the illusion of not having those strong angles on the side of your face, draw the onlooker's eye to the center of your face instead.

As you can't do much to your nose, highlight your lips! Plump it up and make it juicy-looking. Apply gorgeous bold color in cream, then finish off with gloss on the center of the lower lip.

For Round Face

The round face is characterized by a broad forehead, wide cheeks, and a rounded jawline. This face shape is often elongated with a layered shoulder-length haircut that is kept straight at the ears and with volume around the temples.

- Draw attention away from the sides of your cheeks by using the shading technique mentioned above. To slim down your face, use a deeper foundation tone in the hollows of your cheeks. Blend well with a sponge.

- A round spot of blush on the apple of your cheeks will only make you look rounder. Instead, apply the blush or bronzer just underneath your cheekbone in an upward stroke toward your temples. Again, blend well!

- Highlight your eyes and lips. They often appear small against the big space of a round face. Smudge eyeliner on your eyes – never use fine lines. Use dark eye shadow on the outer corners of your eyelids and go light toward the inner corners. This will make your eyes appear wide open and proportionate to your face. For the lips, go for deep or bright colors (according to your skin tone), adding a dab of gloss on the lower lip's center.

Oblong Face

The oblong face is characterized by an almost perfect oval, except that it is a little too long. This face shape is often shortened or widened with bangs or a short bob that stops at the chin.

- Highlight your chin and cheekbones with an illuminator or bronzer.

- Extend your eyebrows toward your temple to create an illusion of width.

- Try for a cat-eye look using your eyeliner. Play with different eye shadows. Go for dramatic, volumized eyelashes. Any or all of these will draw attention to your eyes rather than the length of your face.

For Heart-Shaped Face

The heart-shaped face is characterized by a pointed chin and strong cheeks and jawline. This face shape usually looks best with bangs or a straight cut that slopes down to the shoulders or chin.

- Fine, straight eyebrows with a nice arch will slim down the forehead and balance the rest of the face.

- Use contouring to give the illusion of width on your chin area. Apply concealer or highlighter horizontally on your chin and blend well. This subtle line of light will make your chin appear less pointed.

- Heart-shaped faces often come with strong cheekbones. Too much blush will just make the cheekbones look even more prominent, so go light on the blush or bronzer.

- The Oval Face is considered perfect for its proportions and requires no special corrections. Cheekbones and chin are not pronounced, and the width of the face is usually half the length.

- Emphasize the cheekbones by applying the blush obliquely, and darken the chin and forehead with bronzer.

- If you have short eyebrows, try to make them appear longer and angle the brows down towards the ear lobe.

- The brow pencil is used to darken your eyebrows, not thicken them! That's a mistake you don't want to spend time correcting if you're in a hurry. Use the brow pencil with a light hand, and then blend it in with an eyebrow brush.

Tips for Beautiful Cheeks

Don't neglect your cheeks. Be sure to always apply a little blush or bronzer on them to give your face a full, glowing, and healthy look. Always remember that your health is in the brightness of your eyes and the color of your cheeks.

Cheeks are fairly easy to treat. Here we discuss a technique to help girls with round faces - we have great cheeks.

Buy a cheek trio or a quartet of neutral pinks or plums, depending on your skin tone. Just like an eyeshadow palette, a cheek palette will have a dark, medium, and light shade.

Find your cheekbones. When you smile, you'll notice your cheeks rounding out under your eyes. That's the apple of your cheeks, or your cheekbone.

Now apply the darker shade just below this apple/cheekbone. Blend well with the brush or your fingers. Do not apply the blusher beyond the outer corner of the eyes.

Apply the medium shade on top of the darker shade. Blend, blend, blend, blend. You don't want streaks or smudges. If you only have one shade of blush, you probably already have an idea of how to mimic the different shades. Just apply more below the cheekbone and less above the initial strokes. This gives depth to your cheeks, making your face appear less round.

The lighter shade acts as a highlighter, which should be applied above the middle shade and not too far from the space under your eyes. This method highlights your face and gives you a glow, rewarding you with a slimmer, more youthful appearance.

Elegant Nose Tips

Our noses can be quite problematic at times. They shine at us and they can be too big. But pretty noses make pretty faces: just look at the statistics of nose jobs being done and the income of the cosmetic surgeons who perform them! But don't worry, your nose probably isn't as bad as you think, and I think we've already agreed on the miracle makeup can achieve.

Here's what you can do to make your nose look smaller, more delicate, and generally fabulous.

- **You need two shades of foundation.** One that is two shades darker than your skin and one that matches your skin. Using a sponge or a brush, apply the darker foundation down the length of the sides of your nose, from between your eyebrows, and on downward. Blend, blend, blend.

- **Contour.** Contouring can have negative connotations, thanks to infamous and sensational actresses, but really, contouring is simply adding dimension to your face. You've already seen its power in making your face less round. It can do the same to your nose. Apply your matching foundation over the dark one, down the bridge of your nose, and you'll see how great your nose will look.

- **Mattify.** Always. Shine can make your nose look bigger, so avoid those shimmery effects. Dust your nose with powder to set the magic you just did, and maintain your matte look throughout the day.

- **You can contour your nose with a bronzer.** I recommended having two colors of foundation at the start of this book: one that matches your skin tone and one for when you have a tan. What if you're already tanned? The "darker" foundation would thus be useless, right? So, don't be afraid to use a bronzer!

- If all these steps are too much of a bother for you to do, and you'd rather spend time doing your eye makeup, well then, you don't have to work on your nose to make it look smaller. Highlight your cheeks instead! Glitter blush can detract attention from your nose, creating the illusion that it is smaller than it really is.

- As with cheeks, shimmery and splendid lips can draw attention away from your nose. But pick one spot for the shimmer. Shimmery cheeks and lips are too much together on one face.

CHAPTER 26:

Your Hand And Nails

Nails can be a clue to your overall health. For example, pale nails may indicate anemia. If your nails look green, it could indicate a bleeding ulcer or another internal bleeding. Flaking or brittle nails may indicate a deficiency of iron, calcium, zinc, vitamin A, B6, or B12. Yellow nails may be caused by dark nail polish, smoking, or lung disease.

Proper nutrition can strengthen and soften nails. Be sure to eat a balanced diet that includes plenty of fruits and vegetables, protein, and healthy fats. Taking vitamin and mineral supplements can also help.

Don't soak your nails to soften cuticles, as water causes nails to split and peel. Instead, massage the nails and cuticles with olive or coconut oil. Once the cuticles have been massaged and softened with the oil, push the cuticle back. Do not cut the cuticles, as they protect the nails from infection.

Protect and moisturize your hands and nails. Have lotion in every room of your home to remind you to moisturize. Also, wear gloves when doing household chores to protect your hands and nails.

Tips for Beautiful and Nails

Exfoliate Hands Before Bed

As you get ready for bed, exfoliate your hands. Rub damp hands with a baking soda paste to remove dry skin, diminish wrinkled knuckles and prevent future age spots. Next, apply a moisturizer or massage your hands with coconut oil. If you wear pretty rings and bracelets that draw attention to your hands, you'll want them to look great.

If You Bite Your Cuticles or Nails

Consider getting a manicure from a professional. If you've paid for a professional manicure, you'll be less likely to bite your fingers. You'll be able to match the shade if you bring your own polish to your manicurist if you chip a nail.

Permanent Nail Solutions

If you find that a regular manicure starts to look ratty after a few days, perhaps a more permanent manicure is what you need. You can choose from acrylic nails, gels, and silks.

- **Acrylic Nails**

If you opt for acrylic nails, your manicurist will mix a liquid with a powder and brush the mixture onto your nails, covering the entire nail. This product hardens when exposed to air. The nail is then shaped. Acrylics last up to a month, but gradually the nails will grow out. You must then return to the salon to have your nails filled. The manicurist will file the edge close to the nail bed and then fill in the empty area. If you decide to remove the acrylics, the manicurist will soak your hands in nail polish remover for about 15 minutes.

- **Gel Nails**

Gel nails are similar to nail polish in consistency. They are applied to the nails with a brush. To cure or harden the product, the nails must be exposed to ultraviolet light for up to 2 minutes after each coat. Gel nails, like acrylic nails, wear out over time, and you will need to refill them every 2-4 weeks. To remove the gels, the manicurist will soak the nails in nail polish remover, or the technician can use nail-sized wraps filled with nail polish remover to loosen the artificial nails enough to remove them.

- **Silk Nails**

Silk nails are fabric liners that are glued to weak or damaged nails to help them grow. Silk is used in some wraps, but linen, paper, and fiberglass are also used. The manicurist will mold the material to the shape of the nail, hold it in place and then apply the glue. Over the glued fabric the polish is applied.

These nail treatments really require professional application. Homemade products are difficult to apply and specialized equipment is needed. Be sure to ask your manicurist about proper care between visits, and return to the salon if you want your nails removed. Don't forget to go au naturel from time to time to give your natural nails a break.

Nail Polishing Tips (Manicure and Pedicure)

Gather the right ingredients for a flawless, long-lasting manicure. To prevent polish from chipping or flaking, apply a thin coat of base coat and two thin coats of polish. Finish with a thin coat of quick-drying polish. To make your manicure last, apply a thin coat of quick-drying polish every other day.

To prevent bubbles from forming in the polish, don't shake the bottle. Instead, roll it between your palms. Before applying the polish, wipe your nails with alcohol to remove any oil residue.

The Right Shape and Color for Your Nails

On the hands of older people, shorter, well-groomed nails look better than longer ones. They also make ordinary actions, such as picking things up or typing, easier. Avoid square-cut nails. The best shape is a round oval. Many older women choose polishes in nude or brown shades, but these sometimes don't look good on older skin. Instead, choose a strong, transparent shade or a bright shade. Many prefer the classic French manicure, which looks great at any age.

CHAPTER 27:

Your Clothing: Overview

Clothing is sometimes synonymous with style; at least, we'd like it to be. Style is something every beautiful girl has. For some, it's intuitive; for others, it requires careful study. There are three basic styles that pretty girls tend to go for. These styles are classic, feminine, and elegant. If you don't like these styles, can you still be beautiful? Of course, you can. But if you choose one of these styles and incorporate it into a style you already like, it will be easier to look beautiful.

Classic style is all about restraint. It's all about simple lines and traditional colors. You won't find any 80's neon in these closets. These girls tend not to follow trends unless a trend becomes a classic, and this takes time. They like to wear well-cut clothes that flatter the lines of their natural shapes, and they want to wear natural fabrics. There is nothing frivolous or frugal about classic style.

Do you have to choose one of these styles to be a real pretty girl? No, but it won't hurt you if you do. Once you pick a style, try to make all your future clothing purchases fit the kind of pretty girl you'd like to be. There's always crossover, of course. You can be classic and elegant and also give a touch of sophistication. You can go for romantic or glamorous, which fits well with feminine or elegant styles. You can use a bit of chic in your classic style or add an arty or bohemian touch to feminine or classic.

The styles you least want to wear are punk, flamboyant, western, gothic, or rocker. Can you infuse these styles into yours and still look pretty? Yes, but be careful not to go overboard. If you're into western, use touches on your outfit, like a western bracelet or belt buckle. Don't go overboard unless you're going to be line dancing. If you wear these styles exclusively, you may get into cartoon territory, and your beauty won't be taken as seriously.

The style to be most careful with is the athletic style. Athletic-style clothing is only meant for the gym. There has been an infusion of lazy girls wearing these styles outside of the gym because the clothes are comfortable. Clothing manufacturers have sold them a bill of goods saying it's okay to look lazy. But these clothes are never for pretty girls unless they are actually in the gym, running, or working out. Athletic wear is often not as flattering as other styles, making it look like no effort has been made. Sweatpants away from the gym say that girls have given up on life and don't care about how they look. There's a big difference between looking like you haven't put in much effort and looking like you haven't put in any effort at all. If you see a pretty girl in those clothes, she is pretty despite the clothes and not because of them. Can you imagine how much prettier she would be if she only wore pretty girl clothes?

Another lovely way to style yourself is to pick an influential decade in fashion and take a cue from it. Some of the great decades for clothing were the thirties, forties, fifties, and sixties. Look up these fashions and find examples of feminine, elegant or classic styles and use them with a modern twist. A word of warning, though: never wear a style from a decade that you can remember. This will make you age faster than progeria. You'll look like you went out of style a long time ago and never updated your look. If you're a fan of the eighties and you remember it, you can't wear that stuff and look good.

Knowing Your Positive Traits

It is imperative that you know your positive traits and exploit them to the fullest. Beautiful girls always accentuate the positive. They know what their most fabulous traits are and put the focus on those things. Think you don't have any great traits? Then look for more. You have them, I promise you. Everyone has something that other people wish they had.

Maybe you're thin and clothes fit you well. Maybe you have a nice rack. Maybe your hair is like spun gold or rich silk. Maybe you have a tiny waist. Maybe your skin is smooth and beautiful, your teeth are white and straight, or you have a megawatt smile. Maybe you have deep-set eyes or heart-stopping eyelashes. Maybe your legs are long and toned. Find what you love most about yourself and bring it out.

A great way to make your clothes look fabulous is to have a tailor on hand. When you find an affordable tailor you can trust, put him or her on speed dial. This is your tailor's job: to turn those clothes that only more or less fit you into the clothes of your dreams.

The tailor's job is to help you accentuate the positive and make the clothes fit you as if they were made for you, and essentially, they are being made for you. You don't know what a big difference a good tailor makes. They can make the waistline right at your slimmest point to make you look slimmer. They can loosen the bust so the fabric falls in a flattering way. They can create garments that are the perfect length for you.

For example, the most flattering length for a dress is just below the knee. Ideally, it should touch just where the calf begins so that it gains volume just below the knee. This makes your legs look shapely and your torso look the right height and proportion.

One of the dresses that always seems to work on many girls is the fit and flare style. These dresses are fitted at the bust and looser at the waist. If you have a nice figure, the focus will be on that. Maybe your body is thicker than you would like. The flounce will disguise that and make you look more feminine. Likewise, if you are slim all over, this style will still look pretty on you, confirming that your bust is more important than your waist, no matter how petite the girls are. Of course, I recommend you wear a push-up bra to get the most out of this style, but it will still look lovely if you wear it to go slightly boyish but still feminine.

Another rule of thumb: Always wear a fitted top with a flowy bottom or a closed bottom with a flowy top. Sometimes you can get away with it if you're going to a concert or a dinner party, but never wear a flowy top and a flowy top at the same time. This flowy will make you look like you're wearing a sack (it doesn't flatter anyone) and that you have no idea what you're doing fashion-wise. However, a pair of skinny jeans with a flowy top is cute and trendy. A flowy skirt with a fitted top will accentuate your bust and detract from generous hips. Keep this fashion rule in mind.

Swimwear

For swimsuits, ruching is highly recommended. It hides all imperfections and makes you look more boiled. Try to avoid two-pieces unless you know how to wear them. The most flattering two-piece styles, according to Cindy Crawford, are fitted triangle tops with elastic tie bottoms. Anyone who can pull off a bikini can sport this style.

For one-piece swimsuits, I also recommend shapewear. Walmart has an excellent and affordable line called Suddenly Slim, which is a shapewear and swimsuit in one. You will be amazed at how you look in these styles. There are other more expensive designers, such as Jantzen, that also make shaping swimsuits. If you can find a push-up swimsuit, get one. A larger bust will always make your waist look smaller.

CHAPTER 28:

Your Clothing: Dressing According To Your Body

Identifying your body type is an essential step in building a positive body image. Most of the time, we try to dress a certain way and then end up disappointed because certain clothes don't fit the way we want them to.

The main reason is that we don't dress in a way that flatters our physical build.

We don't all have the same build, so we can't all wear the same type of clothes. Understanding your body structure will help you improve your ability to dress.

Apple

The apple has a round body structure with a heavy middle portion.

This is a complex body type to dress due to the circular structure. However, this does not imply that there are no flattering cuts at all for your body type. Some highlights make your body look great when they are shown. For instance, the ankles and chest area are the best part of your physique.

Dressing Tips

• Wear skirts that are flat in the front.

• A small wedge heel works wonderfully to showcase your ankles.

• Wide-legged denim trousers are perfect for your body type.

- Avoid regular denim with unflattering cuts.

- Avoid dresses with pleats or gathers in the front.

- A balloon top or dress is an absolute is a big No!

Hourglass

The Hourglass has a feminine structure with a slim waist. The upper half is proportionate with the lower half of the body.

Dressing Tips

- Wear fitted tops

- Necklines like a deep V are very flattering.

- Pencil skirts look good.

- Do not hide any part of your physique.

- Replace stilettoes with peep toes and rounded shoes for a more flattering shape.

Skittle

In the Skittle's body, the upper half of the body is slender. The lower half is dramatically wider than the torso.

The idea with this body type is that you need to balance the upper body with the lower body.

The good news is that this body type is much easier to camouflage your lower body.

Dressing Tips

- Vertical patterns are flattering and will make your thighs look slim.

- Broad lapels on your overcoats are a great idea as they draw attention to your torso and shoulders.

- High chunky heels are significant for this body type.

- Avoid patterned pants with loud colors and patterns as they draw attention to your thighs.

- Shirts with a closed collar or polo neck will also make your torso appear more petite than usual.

Vase

The vase-shaped body structure is an elongated version of the hourglass. The bottom is flatter compared to an hourglass. The torso is also flattering.

Dressing Tips

- A wide scooped neckline is excellent for you.

- Use shoes with a nice curve. Stilettoes are your best bet.

- A jacket with a single button will accentuate your waist, which is your narrowest area.

- Do not wear loose clothes.

- Any garment that draws attention to your hip area must be avoided.

- Horizontal stripes around the tummy area can be avoided too.

- Do not wear shoes that are stubby and chunky as they make your legs look shorter.

Cornet

In Cornet, the body has a straight silhouette with wide shoulders. The frame is athletic and tomboyish.

Dressing Tips

- Wear a draping dress that will hug your body in all the right places.

- Skinny jeans will make your waist look slimmer.

- Choose heels that are delicate to highlight the calves and ankles.

- Avoid baggy pants.

- Do not wear t-shirts with a sporty look all the time.

- Monochromes are boring and unflattering.

The Lollipops

In the lollipops body structure, the torso is well endowed, and the waist is short. Legs and lower bodies are slender.

Dressing Tips

- Wear clothes that have gathered around your waist.

- Bell bottoms work well to make your top look less heavy.

- Wear slim shoes to add to the length of your legs.

- Avoid short-sleeved tops.

- Tops that are too tight are definitely unflattering.

- A high waist can make you look extremely disproportionate.

Column

The body is tall in structure. The height is more than the average woman

Dressing Tips

- Gathering and pleats on the tops can break from your monotonous frame.

- Shoes should have good balance and support.

- Choose dresses with a feminine shape to soften the frame.

- Avoid clothes that end at your ankle as they just look like they do not fit.

- Loose and baggy clothes are unflattering.

- Do not invest in chunky shoes.

Bell

The bell body has a round bottom. The top is not exactly slender, but it is smaller in comparison to your base.

Dressing Tips

- Make the shoulders look broader with funnel-shaped coats.

- Kaftans that skim your thighs are very flattering.

- One heel is perfect to balance out the lower body.

- Waistlines with elastic are the most unflattering thing you can think of.

Goblet

The torso of a Goblet body is heavy and square. The stem is exceptionally slender and elegant. The tummy and the breasts are generous.

Dressing Tips

- Deep V necks will accentuate your chest area while making it appear sleek and slender.

- Skirts that are fitted with top strokes are perfect for highlighting your slim and svelte legs.

- Pants with a flaring hemline will balance your top.

- Wear thick heels that are relatively high to enhance your shape.

- Wide and scooped necks are unflattering for your body type.

- Bell sleeves never look good on this body type.

- Tight shirts will only draw attention to your upper half, which is the problem, so to say.

Cello

A Cello body has broad shoulders. The top is heavy. The waist and hip region are wide.

Dressing Tips

- Skirts with a down panel look good.

- Shoes that can support the size of your body will make you look uncomfortable.

- Accentuate your ankles with wedge heels.

- Avoid any ruffles on the top.

- Wear V necks that give you the best shape.

- Large prints and pleats that are concentrated on one area are unflattering.

- Avoid straight cuts and tightly fitted garments as they will draw attention to the problem areas.

Pear

In pear body, most of the weight is distributed on the ballooning thighs with apparent saddle bags. The calves and ankles are not defined like most body types.

Dressing Tips

- Wear trousers with a flat front.

- Straight boots will cover your stubby legs.

- A coat or dress with a belt will accentuate the waist and make you look slimmer.

- Avoid trousers that have a side pocket.

- Pleated skirts make you look wider than you want.

- Bell bottoms or printed pants should always be avoided with a vengeance.

The Brick

The brick body looks very masculine from the back. The buttocks are flat. The waist is not defined with straight legs. Shoulders are vast and athletic.

<u>Dressing Tips</u>

- Wear tops with a sequined band or some feminine detailing around the neck.

- Fish cut skirts with asymmetric prints work well.

- Choose shoes with rounded toes and a pointy heel.

- Avoid clothes with a masculine cut.

- Straight cuts are not the best idea for your body type.

- Avoid shoes with bulky heels as they make your legs look shorter and flatter.

CHAPTER 29:

Your Clothing:
Dressing According To Occasion

C hic and stylish means that you are not only well-dressed, but also properly dressed. Imagine going to a wedding in expensive jeans and a designer top. You'd be labeled as the worst dressed, even more than the poor girl who showed up in a frumpy dress that doesn't suit her.

Here's a complete guide on what to wear to the most common occasions you're likely to attend in your lifetime.

Wedding

Unless specified, weddings are always a semi-formal celebration requiring cocktail dresses in comfortable fabrics. Beading and sequins don't work for daytime weddings or even evening weddings. You should opt for simple but elegant, with embellishments in the same fabric or chiffon. Leave the glitter for the bride. Choose understated silk or silk blends, which also work if the event is of the formal type, regardless of the style of your dress.

Can you wear your dress with straps? Ask the bride, maid of honor, or mother of the bride. Black and red are pretty attention-grabbing colors. If you want to stand out a bit from the inevitable pastel tones, wear jewel tones - red, eggplant, sapphire, or emerald.

In any case, pastel colors are best for daytime weddings, as these are usually held in spring and summer. More intense colors look great for evening weddings or weddings held in autumn and winter in heated ballrooms or cottages.

Are you invited to the ceremony? Places of worship have different protocols. It's always wise to have a shawl ready if you're wearing something strapless - hats are trés chic! But keep it simple. Don't outshine the bride or the mother.

Are you invited to the rehearsal dinner? Save your best for the big occasion. Where is the dinner being held? Restaurants are easy. Dress accordingly, as if you're going to dinner. Wear something you would wear for a first date: something that looks effortlessly stunning.

Job Interview

Whatever you do, self-confidence is important. Be punctual. Also be professional, respecting the expected dress code, or simply looking presentable to the hiring manager.

While a crisp, classic suit goes a long way, today it is no longer the only option. Sometimes it may even be the wrong choice. Know the company if it doesn't provide a dress code. Look on the website; there are bound to be photos of the staff. What do they look like? Mixed, but with a very special touch. You're not with them yet but expect to be. However, offices and large, traditional firms still consider a suit the standard. It says you're serious and determined to get the job.

Be mindful of the position: if you're applying for a creative or artistic job, show your creativity in what you wear. Hiring managers will get a first impression of your ability for the position from your appearance. Jobs in design, media, retail, and technology are booming, competition is fierce and only the smartest make it to the top. Show your intelligence.

Dating

When you go on your first date, you can wear something simple but stylish. Keep it mysterious.

To avoid wardrobe panic, arrange something casual. Go to a place with a relaxed atmosphere rather than a formal restaurant. If you're not sure of the ambiance of the place, go on Google and do a little research to determine what the appropriate style would be. You don't want to go overboard with a dress meant to knock your date's socks off. Choose something comfortable that you've worn before. The first date is not the time to try a new dress or style. Your style is influenced by your personality, so let it shine. Don't try wearing something you wouldn't normally wear. This will only send mixed messages and confuse your date.

If your date insists on impressing, wear something feminine and modest, such as a wrap dress or a soft jacket and skirt combination. Be attractive and leave plenty to the imagination. If your LBD/LDD is rather "gratifying" in terms of the amount of skin you show, don't wear it. LBDs/LDDs are for special dates, much later.

Gala Dinner

As with weddings and meetings with prospective in-laws, educate yourself on appropriate attire. It's better to be informed than wrong. What happened to the dinner? What's the reason for the celebration? You don't want to be overdressed and humiliate your host or anger your colleagues by being overdressed.

Birthdays are usually informal affairs unless otherwise specified. It also depends on the venue and the age of the honoree. In the case of anniversaries, from the age of 20 onwards, it usually goes from semi-formal to formal.

Still not sure? Play it safe with a blouse and skirt combination of good fabric, with modest but nice heeled shoes or boots (depending on the time of year). Keep some nice earrings, a necklace, or a scarf in your purse in case you need to spruce up in a pinch.

Corporate Dinner

Formal events require formal attire. Either way, remember that you're between bosses and clients. You want to be taken seriously and still be seen as a professional, not a "naughty kitten". Keep things nice but modest. Provocative clothing is unprofessional.

Your work attire can go straight to a business dinner, as long as your workplace is not overly casual. You can swap your subtle jewelry for chunky, dangly jewelry and your work shoes for metallic heeled sandals.

LBDs or LDDs are great for company parties, as long as they are not too small (at a minimum, hemlines should reach at or just above the knee). But cover up if your dress is sleeveless or strapless.

The same goes for company picnic parties. Jeans are fine, but not ripped jeans. Shorts are fine, but not too short and not the kind you wear for a day at the beach with the family. Summer dresses are fine with wedge sandals. Once again, nothing strapless and impudent.

Christenings and Other Religious Events

Wear something modest but not boring, and pretty but conservative, to be safe. Choose closed-toe shoes instead of sandals, and keep your shoulders and chest covered. This still leaves you with a lot of options, doesn't it?

Going respectful doesn't equate to going too somber. You're going to a celebration, not a funeral.

Knee-length day dresses are fine for most Christian churches, with or without sleeves. But Jewish synagogues require you to cover up. If you're going to a bar or bat mitzvah celebration right afterward, put a shawl or jacket over your dress and take it off for the party. If there is time in between, you can change. Wear a skirt or pantsuit for the ceremony and party for the festivities afterward.

During Work

Your clothes say a lot about you. At work, you want to be taken seriously, but still maintain your style and feel good about yourself. The workplace is not the right environment to try something daring. Keep it simple and professional. A knee-length skirt with a simple black turtleneck or short-sleeved blouse is ideal. Choose a sensible pair of shoes, such as pumps with a heel of no more than 10 cm. A black, beige, or other neutral-colored pants can also work. Avoid showing too much skin. The hemline should reach the knee or just above. Feminine suits are very elegant and convey confidence.

Going to the Beach

You want to enjoy your weekend at the beach without worrying about wrinkles in your dress or pants. A flirty, flowy summer dress made with a fabric designed to be wrinkle-free is perfect. For dinner out, take a pair of wedges to wear with your dress. Comfortable sandals that are easy to slip on and off are a must. You'll also want to pack a warm knit sweater to protect you from chilly nights. Walking on the beach in jeans and a simple but feminine t-shirt is the ideal outfit. Remember to bring a windbreaker.

Shopping

Shopping is a sport in every sense of the word. It is advisable to wear something very comfortable, even your shoes. The best option is lace-up shoes, so you can easily take them off and put them on to try on new shoes. Wear loose-fitting clothes that you can take off quickly in the dressing room. Avoid collared shirts and clothes with many buttons. A skirt is preferable, as it allows you to try on jeans or tops without too much trouble. Choose tops or pants in neutral colors that match everything you try on. Keep accessories to a minimum.

Going to the Movies

Movie theaters are not the ideal place for long dresses. The hemline drags and can get stained by a spilled drink. Choose a good pair of pants or jeans that you feel comfortable in while seated. Wearing something excessively tight in the waist is not a good idea. If you want to wear a dress or skirt, make it rather casual and with a hemline that reaches your knee when you are standing. A maxi dress is perfect. A warm and comfortable sweater is also perfect to keep the chill of air conditioning away. Leggings paired with a long t-shirt or cardigan and heels are stylish and perfect for sitting in the theater.

CHAPTER 30:

Your Accessories:
Types Of Fashion Accessories

When choosing your accessories, you have to take into account the overall image of your outfit and what you want to achieve with it, as well as the occasion on which you are going to wear it. Accessories should be an extension not only of your outfit, but of your personality.

Jewelry

Jewelry is the most important accessory, so the next chapter will be entirely dedicated to this topic. Jewelry is a personal and unique choice for your personality. Therefore, you should choose your jewelry selectively and wisely.

Accessories for the Head

Hair accessories have survived throughout the ages. New styles have emerged and old favorites are constantly redesigned to suit the latest fashion.

It is very important to wear hair accessories that complement your outfit. If you are representing a certain style, choose accessories in that style as well. With the wide variety of hair accessories out there, there is sure to be an item on the list that suits your outfit.

The most popular hair accessories are bobby pins and clips. Clips come in all shapes and sizes, from large jaw clip to small jaw clips and crocodile clips. Depending on the length of your hair, clips can be used to hold your hair together and out of your way, or you can use them to do updos.

The headband is also a favorite. They are available in hard or soft options. The hard headband usually goes only from ear to ear on the head, while the soft material bands wrap around the head. The bands should fit comfortably. If it hurts, it is too small, and you should buy a larger one.

Scarves can be worn as a head accessory and are very versatile. They can be worn as bandanas, rolled and wrapped around the head like a headband, or they can be worn to cover the head and hair. This is very practical when going out, but you have to keep the style in place.

Another option is hats. Hats are back in fashion in various designs. There are baseball caps, golf caps, and cowboy hats, just to name a few. Hats with wide brims and caps are good for providing extra protection from the sun. Hats are great accessories for themed parties and events to complete the intended theme.

Belts

Belts can be a very important part of your attire. Belts are accessories and should not be worn as a necessity. Belts are there to highlight a slim waist or create the illusion of a slim waist if you have a straight body type.

If you're not sure how to wear a belt, here are a few guidelines:

1. Determine where to wear the belt, where it suits you best. It can be at the waist, just above the waist, or around the hips.

2. Next, you should consider the width of the belt. If you have a long waist and upper torso, wear a wide belt. A slim belt is preferable for someone with a small waist.

3. Belts look good when worn over a dress or shirt. Coordinate the color of the belt to blend in with your clothes. Wear a black belt to create contrast with any color for a dramatic effect or a silver belt for a more romantic look.

4. The material which the belt is made of can also play a role in your confidence. Elastic belts are very flexible and comfortable as it adjusts to your body. If a belt becomes uncomfortable, you will be more aware of it and will draw more attention to it as you constantly try to adjust your belt.

5. Getting used to wearing a belt takes a little time. Get to know yourself and your style. When you find your style, you will be able to wear a belt with confidence.

Scarves

Scarves are fun accessories that can be worn year-round, not just in winter. No one can argue with the extra warmth that scarves provide during the winter. There are many ways to wear fashionable scarves to complete any outfit.

For a stylish look, wear a scarf in the same color as your outfit when wearing a neutral color. Add a garment or two in a different shade to break up the monotony of a single color. Mix different textures to give your outfit even more dimension. For example, you can wear a wool scarf with a woven top.

A scarf is worn around the neck, which will almost immediately draw attention to your face. For this reason, you should wear a color that suits your skin tone and the season. It can add color and warmth to a simple outfit. It can make your outfit look more playful yet elegant when you drape a shawl or scarf over one shoulder and wrap it around your neck.

Don't stick to plain scarves. Be brave and try printed scarves. The scarf should match the main color of your outfit.

Handbags

It is very rare to see a woman in public without some kind of handbag. This is because handbags are used as carrying items so that you can carry your most important items everywhere you go. It has become a necessity and not always an accessory. Here are some ideas to keep it as a necessity but make it look like an accessory.

You can carry the bag over your shoulder, under your arm, or slung across your body. You will need to adjust the length of the strap to the size of the bag. The bag should be in proportion to your figure, so you need to adjust the strap to place it in the right proportion to your body. Wearing the bag under the arm or at the elbow will make your upper body stand out. If you have a large bust, carry a small bag under the arm, or carry the bag lower. The same principle applies to the waist and lower body. Avoid large bags in an area where you don't want to stand out or balance that area with a small bag.

Bags can be any color and don't have to be the same color as your clothes. However, be careful not to carry a bag in a color that clashes with your outfit. Choose a color that matches another key item in your outfit, or carry a neutral bag that works with any color.

If the bag's straps are too short to carry over your shoulder, carry it over your arm or in your hand. The bag should also not hide your clothes at any time. This means that even when you take something out of the bag, it should not spoil your shirt or dress. Rather opt for a clutch or a smaller bag if your purse overwhelms you.

Sunglasses

Sunglasses are a fashion statement for many people, who come to insist on wearing only certain designer brands. Regardless of the brand of sunglasses, the primary function is and should always be to protect the eyes from the sun's harmful rays.

When choosing sunglasses, it is important to make sure that the frame fits the shape of the face. A person with an oval face can wear almost any style of sunglasses, while a square face will look softer with round frames. A person with an elongated face should wear sunglasses with a short frame to shorten the face, and a person with a round face type will look good wearing sunglasses with angular frames.

CHAPTER 31:

Your Accessories: Types Of Jewelry

Jewelry brings beauty to you, your outfit, and your home. It's the most basic of accessories, but it's versatile and easy to incorporate into almost any affair. No matter the occasion, you can find the perfect piece of jewelry to pair with an outfit. With so many options, there's no reason not to have something unique on your wrist or around your neck every day.

Different Kinds of Jewelry

A touch of colored gemstones can add instant glamour to any look. Whether it's emerald earrings, stackable ruby rings, or a necklace with sapphires, every woman should have essential pieces of vibrant stones in her arsenal. Avoid accessorizing overload by wearing a relatively simple necklace over your flashy dresses. Also, your jewelry should be as versatile as possible to avoid drawing too much attention to it. Be careful not to mix jewelry of too many different styles because it's not chic at all. A pearl necklace combined with a huge pair of ethnic and colorful earrings is not a good idea. Simple yet eye-catching, jewelry can breathe new life into basic everyday outfits. **Here are a few jewelry pieces you can try for an instant fabulous look:**

1. **Classic Watch:** Nowadays, watches are more than just an item that tells the time. They have become a status symbol and are often considered one of the many fashion accessories that are necessary for anyone to possess.

2. **Necklace with Pearls:** Pearl necklace can instantly upgrade any look, which is a significant advantage because you won't waste money investing in this for a long time.

3. **Pendant Necklace:** Another timeless piece that you may wear every day is a dainty pendant necklace. Choose a design that best reflects your character, or a memorable event in your life, whether it's a symbol, a number, a word, or a favorite animal!

4. **Dangle Earrings:** Dressy dangle earrings: will definitely add the glam factor to your cocktail dress.

5. **Long-Chain Necklace:** Are delicate and sophisticated. The perfect accessory all year round. Perfect for a casual look if worn in total length.

6. **Diamond Stud Earrings:** Diamonds are a girl's best friend, and the classic diamond stud is every woman's addition to the jewelry collection. The small stones can be worn daily, but they also make for an easy way to look put together in just minutes.

7. **Statement Bracelet:** A bracelet is the most basic piece of jewelry. It's the one you wear every day, so why not make a statement with it? A bold design that has some drama but still feels elegant is perfect for everyday wear.

8. **Charm Bracelet:** Charm bracelets have become very popular recently. They are a great way to commemorate important moments in life because charms can be added for each event. Choose charms that are tasteful and sophisticated so that they will continue to look good over time.

9. **Cocktail Ring:** Cocktail rings are bold and stunning, not only making a glamorous statement but also becoming a talking point at various parties and formal occasions.

10. **Stackable Ring:** Stackable rings have grown in immense popularity in recent years. That means you may wear them individually for subtle, stylish splendor or stack them for maximum impact and a spectacular combination of colors and textures.

CHAPTER 32:

Your Accessories: Accentuating To Style

A ccessories will add an edge to your look. With a few well-chosen pieces, you can turn your new wardrobe into a fashion statement. You'll use your personal style and unique vision to choose the accessories that will personalize your wardrobe.

The key to dressing perfectly with accessories is to follow the advice of your body type. If your body type requires accenting, large necklaces, scarves, and earrings will be your key pieces. Read the tips on your body type and note what and where you need to accentuate, then start shopping.

Accessories can make the difference between a night on the town and an afternoon at the office. Your accessories will help you define your personal style and create several different looks for your favorite outfit. You can take off your bracelets, add some earrings and swap your necklace for a scarf and create a new look without changing your outfit. You don't need to spend a lot of money on jewelry and other accessories. A nice piece of costume jewelry will do the same job as an expensive piece. The point of accessories is to personalize and accentuate, so have fun.

Here are tips for each body type and what accessories work best.

Straight Body

Belts, scarves, and necklaces can help create the illusion of balance by accentuating the bust, neckline, and hips. Look for chunky necklaces, large beads, and anything else that's in style.

If chunky necklaces aren't your thing, try scarves. Look for designs and colors that match more than one item in your wardrobe.

Dark belts that sit at the waist can provide the illusion of a smaller waist, and belts that fall or drape around the hips are perfect for creating the illusion of a thicker topline.

Oval Body

An oval body type should accentuate the neckline and hips and diminish the waist. Since most oval-shaped women have a short neckline, a thick necklace is not the best choice. For this body shape, a necklace with a large pendant is best.

A large pendant will draw attention away from the neck to just above the bust line, accentuating where it is most effective. Scarves may be too much for this body shape, stick with pendants and keep them large, nothing small. To accentuate the hips, try belts that fall or drape around the hips to create the illusion of a smaller waist.

Scoop

The scoop body shape has a smaller bust and larger hips; the key to dressing this body shape is to accentuate the bust line and draw attention away from the hips. This can be achieved with a scarf, a chunky necklace, or a large pendant, nothing small; the point is to draw attention to the bust and cleavage. If you decide to add any scarves, choose colors that accentuate the upper body, nothing drab or bland.

Hourglass Top

For those with a superior hourglass figure, no big necklaces, no bulky scarves, the accentuation should be on the hips and the perfect waist.

Belts that sit at the waist are ideal for showing off a perfect waist, and belts that fall or drape around the hips will accentuate the hips and waist.

Keep necklaces small and opt for bracelets and rings; both rings and bracelets can accentuate the hips and waist because when the arms are down, they fall at the hips and waist.

Hourglass

The key to dressing an hourglass figure is to keep the balance between the top and bottom and accentuate the perfect waist. This can be done in any way you choose.

If you like large or chunky necklaces or scarves, pair them with a draped or draping belt that sits on the hips; this will balance the figure.

If you have smaller necklaces and earrings, pair them with a belt that sits at the waist.

Remember, it's all about balancing your perfect figure.

Inverted Triangle

Accessories for the inverted triangle shape can be achieved by drawing attention to the hips and creating the illusion of balance.

For this body shape, use small necklaces, no scarves, and try belts that drape over the hips and fall downward.

Keep necklaces small and opt for bracelets and rings; both rings and bracelets can accentuate the hips and waist because when the arms are down, they fall over the hips and waist.

Pear

The pear shape has a smaller bust compared to the hips, so accessories at the top are the best choice. Necklaces, scarves, and earrings can draw attention to the top and away from the bottom; this helps balance the shape.

Statement necklaces, chunky pendants, and large pendants work well for the pear shape. Large earrings, such as hoops, will draw attention even higher up and can accentuate the face.

Avoid chunky bracelets or bangles and use small rings, not rings with ornaments or large stones.

Diamond

The diamond shape has a small to medium bust that is larger than the hips with a waist that is larger than the bust line and hips.

A dark belt that sits at the waist can help create the illusion of a smaller waist; this works best with the right jacket to help draw attention away from the waist while the belt works to minimize it.

If you feel uncomfortable with a belt at the waist, look for belts that fall or drape over the hips.

Accentuating the hips also helps to reduce the waistline. Keep necklaces small and opt for bracelets and rings; both rings and bracelets can accentuate the hips and waist because when the arms are down, they fall over the hips and waist.

Some women consider shoes as an accessory; if that's how you see them, you can incorporate different styles into any outfit.

Since your smart wardrobe is created with solid colors, you have a wide variety of styles you can wear with it. Almost any fabric or style will look good with your smart wardrobe.

The accessories you choose will keep your wardrobe on-trend and keep it from looking dated. Shoes are also included in this; fashionable shoes can take a simple outfit to new fashionable heights.

Remember to look for accessories that are trendy and modern; even if you're not into fashion, a modern piece can help you create a fashion statement.

Your new smart wardrobe begs to be accessorized. It's been designed with accessories in mind. Whatever outfit you choose, accessories will add a special touch. The right belt, necklace, and bracelets, or a stunning printed scarf and a drapey belt can add the perfect amount of style and color to your look.

Use the style and colors of accessories to personalize your look. Accessories can make you stand out, blend in and even express your personality. You can use accessories to glam up, go boho or add a touch of class to a simple outfit.

With the right accessories, you can turn your chic wardrobe into a fashion statement that shows off your personal style.

CHAPTER 33:

Your Shoes

B esides having an irresistible appeal to most women, shoes are actually a key accessory to any expensive-looking outfit.

A quality shoe with the most appropriate print for your figure can turn an ordinary outfit into a trendy and fashionable look. With a well-made shoe, you can look stylish and sophisticated even if you are wearing cheap jeans and a plain white T-shirt. On the contrary, if you wear ugly shoes, you can look cheap and sloppy even if you wear designer clothes.

Therefore, quality shoes are a must-have staple for any stylish woman. This does not mean, however, that you can get a luxurious outfit just by choosing any type of shoe in some designer store, as you can find ugly shoes also in the most expensive stores.

Therefore, the right choice is essential to ensure the first-class result without spending a fortune.

Indeed, you can buy shoes of a certain style in some low-budget stores, but ensuring an impeccable result. But some shoes should never be bought in budget stores if you want to achieve an elegant and sophisticated result. I am referring, in particular, to pumps and stilettos, as well as knee-high boots.

These styles require more technical expertise to deliver an impeccable result, and for this reason, it is not easy to find them in a low-priced department store.

However, you're likely to find gorgeous high-end pieces during sales (both in stores and online) and/or at some factory outlets, where you can pick up a great pair of Sergio Rossi stilettos for less than $150.

The colors you choose may not be the most neutral, but don't forget that well-made, brightly colored heels can serve to liven up an all gray, black, or blue outfit, creating a polished and stylish ensemble.

Here are some tips for choosing your perfect heels:

- When shopping for expensive designer shoes, choose only timeless styles. This way, you'll have a stunning piece that will last you for years and always look current, no matter what the trends.

- Furthermore, classical shoe design usually guarantees the most flattering outcome and elongates your silhouette (just think about the ageless bicolor Chanel shoe).

- The most comfortable option for heels is a slightly curved heel placed centrally under the heel of your foot: this design, in addition to making the shoe more comfortable when walking, visually reduces the heel's height, allowing a very proportioned outcome even for those that do not have long legs.

- The softness of the material is essential for perfect comfort. Unfortunately, some very expensive brands use very stiff leather, so be careful in your purchases (and when buying online, be sure that the return is easy).

- For a look that is luxurious and sophisticated, the rule must always be taste and proportion. Therefore, the height of the heel should be proportional to the length of your lower leg. If you are not very tall, remember that—even if you crave very high heels— a heel that's too high will make your legs look shorter by contrast, so if you want a harmonious and chic effect, it's smarter to wear a lower heel.

- For a slimming effect, low-vamp styles and minimal designs are preferable. The more skin you show, the more your legs are visually stretched out.

- Study the design of the "staple production" of top brands. This basic production is usually made of perfect, timeless, and never-changing designs (why change perfection?). If you carefully study any detail, you can then look for similar but more affordable ones elsewhere. And you can spot beyond any possible doubt if the item you're buying is classy or trashy.

Another key item in any woman's closet is a pair of knee-high leather boots. Whether they are low heeled or high heeled, they can easily give your legs a tapered shape while elongating your entire figure and adding class to your entire look.

Since knee-high boots almost completely hide your lower leg, they can be incredibly useful for camouflaging any imperfections of the leg itself (too thin, strong calf, or not exactly slim ankles) and its length (which becomes less noticeable). If you combine knee-high boots with skinny jeans and a coat with a belt slightly higher than the waist, your legs will look longer and slimmer, and your whole figure will look perfectly proportioned (and also very sophisticated).

Also, knee-high boots are a must to give you a sophisticated look when wearing elegant skirts, downplaying any possible excess in the print or colors of the skirt.

For a flawless result, pay attention to a few details:

- One of the most important things to keep in mind when buying knee-high boots is the length of the shaft: for those who do not have very long legs, a shaft can end up being too long, which besides being uncomfortable is not chic. The solution is to look for boots with shorter legs or have your boots shortened by a good shoemaker.

- Top-quality knee-high boots are indispensable when buying high-heeled styles, as pulling off an impeccable heel is not a feature you will easily find with cheaper brands.

- Conversely, with low-heeled designs, you can get impeccable results even with not-so-expensive productions.

Platform pumps shouldn't even be considered. No matter what the trends say. Besides looking cheap, no matter their price or brand, platforms will give your step a heavy, tired sound. You'll look like an overweight miner is approaching, not a sophisticated, chic woman. Forget it.

Knee-high boots should always be genuine leather. Leather boots are not suitable, as the faux leather used on such a large surface is clearly noticeable and has a cheap result (unlike leather summer sandals, whose faux leather straps are thin enough to make the difference almost imperceptible).

By contrast, well-made suede can have a totally satisfactory result, even if it is synthetic.

CHAPTER 34:

Your Underwear

Why don't we think about spending a bundle on gorgeous dresses and gowns and getting our hair, makeup, and nails done for a big night on the town, and then spoil all the effort by wearing the wrong underwear?

And how many times do we go out to buy a dress for a special occasion and don't put on the underwear we'll wear with that dress? Trust me, it's the only way to get a really good idea of how the dress will look. Just like a house needs to sit on a solid foundation, the same goes for your clothes. The foundation is the key to looking your best.

Bras

Many women don't even know what a properly fitting bra can do for them and what a proper fit means. So here are the things you should look for when shopping for the right bra.

1. Your entire breast should be contained within the cup.

2. Your breast tissue should be shaped, separated, lifted, contained, and supported by your bra.

3. Your bra should not dig into your shoulders.

4. The center front of your bra should fit close against your breastbone.

5. You should easily be able to slip a finger underneath the band at the base of the cups.

6. Your bra should not ride up in the front or back.

According to Jan Larkey in her book Flatter Your Figure, "A well-fitting bra should touch the breast at the sternum (cleavage) and support the breast at mid-chest level with no bulges." If your bra hurts, rides up your back, doesn't lay flat against your sternum, or the straps dig in or slide down your shoulders, you have a poorly fitted bra.

As with most garments, there are no uniform sizing standards in the industry. One manufacturer's "C" cup may be another manufacturer's "D" cup, and so on. You should try on many bras to get the best fit. There are two measurements you should consider when choosing a bra. The first is the band size, which is the size of your rib cage, and the second is the cup size, which is the size of your actual breast tissue. Since all women are different, it's impossible to give a definitive rule for everyone when it comes to sizing a bra, but these general guidelines should at least help you get an idea of your size.

To get your band size, measure your rib cage under your breasts while wearing the bra that fits you best, not the one that fits best. Then add five centimeters to the measurement. If you get an odd number, go to the next higher even number.

To calculate your cup size, gently measure around your chest and across your nipples. If the band measurement and the cup measurement are the same, you have an "AA" cup. If the cup measurement is one inch more than the band measurement, you are an "A" cup, and two inches more is a "B", three inches a "C", four inches a "D", five inches a "DD", six inches a "DDD", etc. If the bra doesn't fit your sternum, try a larger cup size.

You can also experiment with fit using the "one size up, one size down" rule. Let's say you have a "38D" bust. You've tried on every "38D" bra you could find and nothing is supportive and comfortable. Try going up to a "40C" or a "36DD". If you go up one size in band width, go down one cup size, and vice versa. (This doesn't always work, but I've seen it work more often than not).

Your bust line should be about midway between your shoulders and waist. Many women think they have a small waist when they just need to get the right bra to lift the bust line into place.

If you are small-breasted, avoid bras with nipple seams. There's no reason to draw attention to what isn't there. If you have a large bust, the best support is provided by underwires. Choose bras with wide straps to help reduce pressure on your shoulders. Women with a short waist also do better with an underwire bra, as it provides more support and helps lift the bust line. Whatever your size, if you're going sleeveless, make sure the armhole of your suit completely covers the bra. Showing your underwear should be reserved for intimate and private moments only.

When deciding which color to buy, choose a white bra to wear under white or light-colored clothing, a black bra to wear under black or dark-colored clothing, and a skin-colored bra to wear under more sheer clothing. Never wear a dark bra under a light-colored top or vice versa. I know you see it in fashion magazines, but trust me, it's not a good look, and no one is going to pay attention to a word you say. They will be totally focused on your bra. If that's what you want, by all means, go for it.

The best way to find a good bra is to have it tried on by an expert. If you're extremely large or small, and your size isn't found in department stores (or there isn't a good selection), try visiting a specialty underwear store, or go to a company that fits bras for mastectomy patients. (Trust me, they really know what they're doing.) Don't clamor for a good bra. Not only does it help your clothes look better, but it can also help reduce the strain on your back if you have a large bust. A good bra really is worth its weight in gold. Gold? Hell, platinum.

All-in-One

All-in-ones are wonderful for lifting your chest and tucking in your tummy. Make sure your garment is long enough so that it doesn't pull your chest down or squeeze your crotch. As for body slimming garments, these gorgeous inventions are wonderful for lifting your bust, tucking in your tummy, and slimming your thighs. Remember that these garments are not meant to take off ten pounds, but to remove any unwanted bulges and create a cleaner line, so don't buy them tight. If you find it uncomfortable, it's probably too small.

Panties

Look for panties that don't ride up in the back or cinch around the tummy or thighs. Don't buy underwear that is too tight. If you wear a lot of pants, buy briefs instead of bikinis. You don't want panty lines showing under your clothes. Gross. Seeing a woman with a panty line under her underwear is a real "NAGL" (Not a Good Look). If you have hip-hugging pants, by all means, buy a pair of bikinis. If not, leave them at the store. The same color rules apply to panties as for bras. If you wear a white skirt or white pants, wear white panties. Undergarments should not show through clothing at any time, regardless of whatever quirky, trendy style some "designer" comes up with.

Girdles

Girdle size is determined by the size of your hips. Measure the widest part of your hips and then measure your waist. Find out the relationship between your waist and hip measurements and then check this relationship against the manufacturer's sizes. Don't wear the girdle too tight. The purpose of a girdle is not to make you look two sizes smaller, but to eliminate bulges and smooth your figure.

Briefs/Camisoles

All women should have at least one-half slip in a nude color to wear under light-colored skirts and one full slip to wear under dresses. If you want to keep blouses from clinging, you should also have a light-colored camisole. White and light blouses, skirts, or light materials can show through in some light, and wearing a camisole or slip creates a cleaner look by keeping the material away from your body.

Hose Down

Make sure you have the right style and color of hose for the outfits you have in your closet. You don't want to give up a good outfit because you didn't remember to buy the right hosiery. Rule of thumb: Never, ever, ever wear black tights with a white or light-colored skirt and never wear white house with a black or dark-colored skirt. I know some women love to wear white tights with a dark dress, but remember that the eye is drawn to light, bright colors before dark ones. If you wear white stockings with a dark dress, the viewer's attention will be focused on your legs instead of your face, which is where it should be. Your stockings should have the same value as your outfit. You will always be safe wearing sheer stockings that let your natural skin color show through.

Don't wear a reinforced toe with an open-toed sandal. And remember that the dressier the shoe, the sheerer the stockings should be; the sportier the shoe, the more opaque the stockings should be. Never wear stockings with a dress or skirt, especially if the dress or skirt has back, front or side slits. It looks very bad.

Spend a little time and money on all your undergarments and you'll be amazed at the difference in your appearance. And with a solid foundation established, you can easily build a gorgeous frame that is you!

CHAPTER 35:

Your Fitness: Do Some Exercise

The Role of Exercise on Your Beauty

Exercise keeps the body in optimal condition so that muscles, bones, and internal functioning remain young and healthy. The best way to look younger on the outside is to make sure you feel young on the inside.

The great thing about exercise is that it's all good for you. There are thousands of different ways to be active, so you can choose the activity or sport that you enjoy the most. The most important thing is to have fun and get your heart rate up for at least 20 minutes a day.

Yoga

Yoga is a great exercise that helps prevent aging. Not only does it improve circulation, but it also strengthens bones and muscles and gives you more flexibility. This will give you better body alignment, which will take years off your appearance. It will also firm and tone your muscles so you don't have to worry about any movement or sagging.

There are plenty of great courses on yoga for all levels of experience. You can get a video to do yoga from home, or you can sign up for a class at your local gym.

Some of the best anti-aging yoga poses are as follows:

- Standing Forward Bend

- Proud Warrior

- Side Stretch

- Tree Pose

- Upward Facing Dog

- Seated Twist

- Bridge Pose

- Reclining Twist

Doing yoga daily can help reduce cellulite and firm your skin. It will keep you looking younger and is extremely healthy for you. It also has countless proven benefits for your mental and emotional state. So yoga is a great all-around treatment that can rejuvenate you in every possible way.

Cardio

Cardiovascular exercise is any exercise that gets your blood pumping. This includes walking, running, swimming, hiking, biking, and other activities where you can feel your heart start to race. Cardiovascular exercises are a great way to look younger because they improve circulation, which makes your skin look radiant and alive. It also makes you feel younger on every level. You feel more energetic, fitter, and ready to take on anything. This will give you a lively, youthful expression as you face your day.

Strength Exercises

Strength exercises are those that focus on muscle development rather than speed, endurance, flexibility, or agility. These are exercises such as weight lifting, squats, or push-ups. If you don't have weight training equipment at home and don't want to go to the gym to lift weights next to dozens of beefy guys, there are some great strength exercises you can perform at home using only your own body weight and common household items.

Strength exercises are a great way to get rid of cellulite and tone your body. Doing strength exercises doesn't necessarily mean you have to become a bulky bodybuilder. You can use them simply to tone and shape your body so that there is no cellulite, no excess flab, and no sagging skin.

Here are some good strength exercises that you can do at home without any other equipment:

- Push-Ups

- Squats

- Lunges

- Triceps Dips

- Dynamic Prone Plank

- Crunches

There are many YouTube videos you can watch online on how to correctly perform those above exercises.

Sports

Sports are one of the best ways to stay active and get enough exercise in your regular routine. Team sports have the added advantage of keeping you motivated because you are part of a team. Individual sports, on the other hand, are better for those who prefer to go at their own pace. Whatever type of sport you choose, you'll usually get a great combination of cardio and strength training. Some of the best sports for staying young are soccer, tennis, swimming, cycling, and golf. Swimming is great for those with weak joints or arthritis, because it has a low impact on the joints while providing a great cardiovascular workout and even building muscle strength (which ultimately might even help your joints!).

Facial Exercises

In addition to physical exercises that rejuvenate your body, you should also do some facial exercises that will keep the skin on your face and neck firm and wrinkle-free. This will make your face look as young as your body. Facial self-massage has many benefits: first of all, it is free, it doesn't cost anything, secondly, it is systematically really effective".

It stimulates circulation and lymphatic drainage, so the immediate effect is a more" deflated "face, clean, without swelling, stagnation, and therefore toxins, instant brightening effect. Then going on to work the facial muscles, long-term firms, and tones the oval fighting against the small sagging caused by the force of gravity.

The skin must be strictly clean, after cleansing and toning. Better not to do the massage "dry", but apply a product on the skin to facilitate the movement of the movements. Ideally with a natural oil.

1. Start by stimulating the lymphatic system: draw small concentric circles on the side of the neck, going from the throat to the ears and backward, from the bottom upwards.

2. To define the profile line: the thumbs point under the chin, the hands fan out: they go up from the chin towards the ears, following the jaw line. The index fingers glide over the cheeks, activating circulation. Next, go over the chin line with gentle pinches made with the thumb and forefinger.

3. Rejuvenate the smile: with open hands and flat fingers, draw small circles on the sides of the mouth, pushing the cheek muscle upward with each step. Proceed with smaller circles only around the mouth, where expression lines and so-called "marionette" lines form, pulling the smile downward.

4. Soften the vertical lines: with the middle finger "go up" from the sides of the mouth along the nasolabials, pushing upwards. You can also continue towards the forehead, passing through the center of the eyebrows and ending at the forehead.

5. Lift the cheeks: with closed knuckles, do gentle push-ups pushing toward the cheekbone from the center of the cheeks.

6. Lift the profile: with hands open and flat, glide from the chin to the temple towards the other, alternating hands continuously, in a quick, continuous motion.

7. For the eye contour, alternate two movements: "stretch" the dark circles with two fingers, from the nose to the ears and follow the line of the eyebrows with your fingers, gently pushing upwards.

8. Against fine wrinkles: finish with a "cris cross" of small zig zags with your fingers. On the temples to minimize crow's feet, on the forehead for expression lines.

9. Last shock: perform quick "push-ups", with the palm of the hand open, from the bottom up and from the center to the outside of the face.

10. Conclude by making small pressures with the fingers still in the hairline, in small circles that release the tension.

More Tips

Explore and try many different types of exercise before you settle on one. This helps you stay motivated because you find a form of exercise that you really like, so you feel like going out and doing it.

Variety is the spice of life: even if you find a type of exercise that you like, don't limit yourself to it. While you're doing that exercise regularly, be sure to try others here and there. Spice up your routine by doing several different types of exercise regularly. Variety will ensure that you never get bored with your routine.

- **Track your progress:** keep a daily log of the exercise you do (and even the foods you eat). Even if you don't have a specific weight or fitness goal you're trying to achieve and just want to keep yourself looking younger, tracking your progress is a great way to stay motivated. You can see how far you have improved since your first workout. This is a huge motivator for those days when you feel like you have sort of stagnated.

- **Know your body:** above all, listen to what your body is telling you. If you are overdoing it on the exercise, you could end up causing serious damage that could leave you bedridden for months. That's months of not being able to exercise, so you will risk falling out of shape again. So if you feel like you have hit your limit, don't try to push yourself past it. The more exercise you perform, the better you will become. Allow your body to improve at its own rate.

- **Exercise with friends or sign up for a class:** a great way to stay motivated to exercise regularly is to do it with others. Find a workout buddy or sign up for a training class at your local gym or recreational center. Having others that you work out with will help you get off your butt on those days when you don't feel especially motivated to exercise.

CHAPTER 36:

Yourself: The Value Of Loving Thyself

We often feel that our attractiveness is a measure of our worth. We spend hours comparing ourselves to other people, dreaming of the day when we look as good as they do. As it turns out, this can be a big mistake. It turns out that self-love and acceptance are some of the most powerful forces for health and happiness, not only for ourselves but also for those around us. Sure, it's good to feel attractive. But what matters most is how you feel about yourself. Until you accept your worth, your confidence will come and go with the flow of others' opinions. You'll spend many hours in front of the mirror trying to improve your appearance, but the truth is it doesn't matter. The most important factor is how you feel about yourself, and the only way to find that is to stop comparing yourself to others who are much more handsome or beautiful than you.

You Can't Improve If You Think You're Already Perfect

Shifting the balance from doing more and squeezing more into your day to doing less and being more self-loving as a super busy working woman you recognize and appreciate the value of more time for yourself and self-love, however, putting it into practice is daunting, especially if you've spent years, like most women, putting the needs, wants and desires of your family before your well-being.

And with that, there's nothing wrong.

In fact, the determination to provide your family with a clean, cared for and safe home is part of your motivation to relentlessly aspire to "do more and cram more into your day." What I mean is, when you have to put on the brakes, look in the mirror and ask yourself "what about me, what do I want?" and turn on the love light to satisfy your desires and shake up your inner core. In many cases, the better you are at seeing life through the lens of self-love and your happiness without feeling guilty and "selfish" for putting yourself first, the more you will practice self-love. Ultimately, all spiritual teachings and doctrines stress the value of self-love and acceptance.

3 Self-Love Activities to Make You Love Yourself More

Write Self-Love Quotes, Affirmations, and Inspirations

Build your affirmations and write them down. You can put your affirmations in your purse as an extra treat for yourself or write them on your phone and read them to yourself during the day, especially when you feel anxious. You will immediately relax into the gentler side of your being.

Pray

If you're not a Christian, you may be confused by the idea of meditating. It's time to appreciate the importance of spending a few minutes in silent contemplation and prayer.

Meditate

If you do meditation, you'll know that it's one of the best gifts. There are plenty of meditations out there, and you will come across different techniques and insights during your path of self-love. As a beginner, studying and acquiring yoga from an experienced teacher is always better. Here is a guide

Self-Love Meditation for You to Practice

Once you've said your three daily affirmations, brewed your morning cup of tea, and said your journal, get comfortable finding a quiet area and set a 3-minute timer on your phone, breathe in and out steadily through your nose, drop your shoulders and read a meditation passage aloud to yourself. Sit quietly after reading it, and take a couple more minutes sitting still before resuming your day when the timer stops.

Finding Your Way to Self-Love

It is the mystery we pose to ourselves as we recover and rebuild our broken self-esteem. We want to respect ourselves more fully and enjoy ourselves. Certainly, we know the anguish of dragging around those old feelings of worthlessness. We even learn how we become more "sensitive" and self-critical.

But how do we come to feel self-love from these feelings of pain and self-denial on earth? How do we value ourselves when we so clearly don't respect ourselves in many ways?

Don't be depressed if you feel this discomfort. Often it will seem that "you can't get there from here" in your search for the path to self-love. This obvious stagnation is to be expected.

And here's why. We must first feel full and nourished to feel happy and have a positive sense of ourselves. Of course, the issue is that these negative feelings of self discourage us from being adequately satisfied and full.

This is especially true since our sense of self, our self-image, our entire personality relies heavily on these wounded emotions. As we "tell" ourselves primarily through this wounding-as not enough (not big enough, not small enough, not accomplished enough, not "complete" enough, etc.)-we rob ourselves of that essential, ongoing nourishment we need to find ourselves more.

So our double bind is there. We can't see our worth to be filled and see our worth; we can't fill ourselves. So how are we supposed to get here?

Fortunately, the Bridge to Self-Love is an intermediate step, a "condition" that bridges the gap between that deficiency state of self-rejection and the normal sense of self-love. It is a place that allows us to continue to nurture ourselves, mindful of self-negative feelings so that we can restore and reawaken the inherent sense of being well and necessary.

And the middle ground is self-acceptance and self-respect. Unlike that mystical and distant land of self-love, it's remarkably easy to find this middle place... And incredibly strong.

Self-acceptance and kindness aren't about trying to convince yourself that you're good or effective (or whatever) the moment your damaged emotions warn you that you're not. And it's not about having to kill yourself and correct what's "wrong" with you to fulfill the intense, perfectionist vision. None of these responses do you much good.

Getting to this middle ground requires nothing more than managing yourself in reaction to these painful feelings and stressful moments with patience and compassion.

Let's be clear. These hurt feelings you don't deny. And you don't doubt that it's difficult. You simply respond in a different way to these painful feelings.

Serving' you' instead of the hurt feelings You're taking a different role'. You're stepping back and realizing that, as intense as these hurt feelings sound, they are just that: hurt feelings. They are feelings that create a hurt place. They don't give you accurate information about your dignity. They only warn you of a wounded position.

And you choose to be compassionate, caring, and healing to yourself first in reaction to that wounded position.

Look again at the difference. You choose to handle yourself with dignity, care, and compassion instead of collapsing into these false and negative feelings about yourself, instead of believing them, seeing yourself as a corrupt person, and driving yourself further. By adding kindness and understanding to this painful place, you react to this painful signal.

Keep in mind that this is not about "fixing yourself" to regain your self-esteem. It is about self-nurturing. Your task is not to please yourself or the "wounded" perception of your life. Your task is to fix the wound that is deep down: to feed the poor point of judgment.

And you do this by coming to this position with patience and compassion rather than harshness.

In fact, a sign of their bruised self-esteem is that determination and hardness to repair themselves. A strict response is a continuation of biting and rejecting behavior.

Therefore, if you choose to treat yourself with calm and compassion instead, you break that self-hardening pattern. Regardless of the terms of what you "know" is wrong with you, when you can step back to continue to be compassionate and embrace yourself, the true meaning within you continues to be nurtured.

It is awakened. Your positive sense of yourself gets stronger and stronger when you follow this strategy.

And just to be sure. Self-acceptance does not discourage you from taking positive steps for your growth and progress. Or to make necessary changes in your life. These efforts require you to be especially understanding, patient, and self-approving. This is the strength you need to recover, improve and move forward.

An RX for those excruciating moments of self-rejection. Needless to say, kindness and empathy probably won't be your primary reaction when that feeling of worthlessness rears its ugly head for the first time. At first, we're going to want to collapse into those painful emotions.

So, when that happens, we need to pull back a bit and remember that these feelings are not accurate. They are hurt feelings that take you to a hurt place. Let the discomfort remind yourself to be kind and healing.

For these difficult moments, give it a drug. And the more sensitive these unpleasant positions become, the more careful, gentle, and cautious you must be with yourself. Furthermore, the challenge we encounter in learning to love ourselves is that particularly painful emotions correlated with damaged self-esteem have the unpleasant ability to "erase" our sense of self-worth and self-esteem altogether... And, in essence, we cannot find love for ourselves.

We need to be prepared for this very "natural" response to our woundedness. And consider it sympathetically.

Patience and forbearance, fortunately, are expressions of kindness. Especially when they are directed at you, and this small movement will begin to bring you back to you immediately: to wholeness and to life.

What are the Signs That You Lack a Love For Yourself?

Check out below the 3 indicators that will alert you whether you lack self-love or not.

- First, ask yourself if you believe that a self-love is an act of selfishness?

- Second, do you need other people around you to praise?

- Third, do you need to make others happy about yourself feeling happy?

Don't hesitate if you lack self-love. It's easy to create. The first move is to realize that you need it.

You can build these strategies to build self-love inside yourself.

- Take care of yourself every day. Remember to do simple things like taking vitamins, eating whole foods, and going out on walks to energize your body. We often get distracted in the hectic day-to-day everyday life by taking care of our jobs, debts, and families, which contributes to gradually forgetting to take care of ourselves.

- Embrace your faults or (short-comings) Let yourself realize that making mistakes is OK. Life is not about being flawless because there is no perfection. It's not hard to learn how to accept yourself, but it requires deliberate reflection and knowing that you're losing it.

- You also have to overcome the shame of prior events. It's helpful to keep in mind the following premise, "I don't regret. no regrets for anything I've ever done." You can't beat yourself up for what you've already done because these things can't be changed. You have to pardon yourself. Be mindful that you are going to make various choices in the future.

Without remorse and without continuing to act involuntarily, you can choose to take full responsibility for your actions. You must agree not to compare yourself to others. Compassion arises from the lack of unrealistic expectations of others.

Soon you will be able to remain for days in states of great joy by accepting people where they are. Not having to change things will take a great deal of internal pressure off you. Acceptance is a condition of non-resistance. It is better to let go, and the experience costs you. There is nothing to avoid because everything is there to support you. It takes years to accept this idea, but if you can do it, it helps. By doing this exercise, you will develop your self-love and learn to appreciate what is in you.

Conclusion

Every woman can quickly and easily identify her figure, but few can reliably pinpoint her assets. To create a comfortable personal style, you need to be able to recognize both strengths and weaknesses. Once you can do that, you'll know how to accentuate the positive and eliminate the negative.

Believe in your beauty. No woman believes she has a perfect body, but a woman who believes in herself has great self-esteem and projects self-confidence. The beauty she sees in herself is inevitably seen by others.

A good fit is critical. Make your clothes fit you. The reason it's hard to find clothes that always fit you great is not that the clothes aren't made for you, but that you haven't had them tailored. Remember that the fashion industry is cutting out the hourglass figure and that 65% of women are triangles. We need to combine comfort with the fit.

Balance and proportion are essential. Always dress to balance your body. For example, if you are short-waisted, wear a long top and a short skirt. If you wear a belt, match it to the color of your top. These tips will help you elongate your waist.

On the other hand, if you have a long waist, wear a short top along with a long bottom, and match the color of your belt to the color of your skirt or pants. This will help shorten the waist. Both concepts help achieve visual balance.

Be confident. Stand tall, with your shoulders erect, and let the world see your inner confidence. Good posture is the number one indicator of good self-esteem.

Do you say you lack confidence? No problem. Here's one of the world's best-kept secrets: Fake it until you make it! Imagine the qualities that a confident person possesses. Assume the posture and characteristics and it won't be long before you're feeling supremely confident. It's true. You can literally build self-confidence if you start emulating the mannerisms of people who already possess great confidence. If you don't believe me, try it. You'll be surprised how fast it works. Confidence is your greatest asset.

Believe in yourself, find reasons to smile every day because your positivity will be your most powerful weapon. Take all the time you deserve to take care of yourself. I wish you that your life will be a source of beauty and joy for you and everyone around you.

Printed in Great Britain
by Amazon

44553915R00116